GASTRIC SLEEVE

The Complete Guide With Delicious Meals to Enjoy Your Weight Loss Diet

(Easy Meal Plans, effortless and Delicious Recipes)

Terry Slater

Published by Sharon Lohan

© Terry Slater

All Rights Reserved

Gastric Sleeve: The Complete Guide With Delicious Meals to Enjoy Your Weight Loss Diet (Easy Meal Plans, effortless and Delicious Recipes)

ISBN 978-1-990334-84-9

All rights reserved. No part of this guide may be reproduced in any form without permission in writing from the publisher except in the case of brief quotations embodied in critical articles or reviews.

Legal & Disclaimer

The information contained in this book is not designed to replace or take the place of any form of medicine or professional medical advice. The information in this book has been provided for educational and entertainment purposes only.

The information contained in this book has been compiled from sources deemed reliable, and it is accurate to the best of the Author's knowledge; however, the Author cannot guarantee its accuracy and validity and cannot be held liable for any errors or omissions. Changes are periodically made to this book. You must consult your doctor or get professional medical advice before using any of the suggested remedies, techniques, or information in this book.

Table of contents

Part 1 1
Introduction 2
Chapter 1: Bariatric Surgeries 5
Chapter 2: A New You 23
Chapter 3: Eating Guidelines For Pre-Op And Post-Op 32
Chapter 4: Early Post-Op Foods 45
High-Protein Milk 45
Pumpkin Spice Latte Protein Shake 48
Double Fudge Chocolate Shake 50
Protein-Packed Peanut Butter Cup Shake 52
Vanilla Apple Pie Protein Shake 54
Tropical Mango Smoothie 56
Chapter 5: Breakfast Recipes 58
Smoothie Bowl With Greek Yogurt And Fresh Berries 58
Cherry-Vanilla Baked Oatmeal 61
High-Protein Pancakes 64
Southwestern Scrambled Eggs Burritos 66
Hearty Slow Cooker Cinnamon Oatmeal 68
Mini Bariatric Sized Meatloaf 70
Chapter 6: Lunch Recipes 72
Bashed Chicken With Tomatoes, Olives, And Capers 72
Gingered Ham 74
Lamb And Crispy Potato Hot Pot 77
Rosti-Style Herder's Pie 79

California Burger 81
Chapter 7: Vegetarian Recipes 83
Roasted Vegetable Quinoa Salad With Chickpeas 83
Mexican Stuffed Summer Squash... 85
Barley-Mushroom Risotto 87
Coconut Curry Tofu Bowl 89
Curried Eggplant And Chickpea Quinoa 92
Chapter 8: Seafood Recipes 94
Tuna Noodle-Less Casserole.. 94
Herb-Crusted Salmon 96
Slow-Roasted Pesto Salmon 98
Lemon-Parsley Crab Cakes 99
Seafood Cioppino...101
Chapter 9: Poultry Recipes 104
Slow Cooker White Chicken Chili..104
Grilled Chicken Wings 106
Ranch-Seasoned Crispy Chicken Tenders 108
Chicken "Nachos" With Sweet Bell Peppers 110
Baked "Fried Chicken" Thighs 112
Chapter 10: Snacks And Dessert..115
Superfood Dark Chocolates...115
Chocolate Chia Pudding 117
Chocolate Brownies With Almond Butter..............................119
Lemon-Blackberry Frozen Yogurt 121
Old-Fashioned Apple Crisp 123
No-Bake Peanut Butter Protein Bites With Dark Chocolate 125

Chapter 11: Sauces And Seasoning 127
Greek Salad Dressing 127
Creamy Peppercorn Ranch Dressing 129
Mango Salsa 131
Perfect Basil Pesto 132
Marinara Sauce With Italian Herbs..134
Chapter 12: Soups And Salads..136
Creamy Chicken Soup With Cauliflower 136
Baked Potato Soup 138
Chicken, Barley, And Vegetable Soup...140
Shrimp Cocktail Salad..142
Tomato, Basil, And Cucumber Salad...144
Chapter 13: Tips For Eating Out 146
Conclusion 148
Part 2 149
Introduction...150
Chapter 1: Why Get Sleeved? 152
Chapter 2: Breakfast 170
Southwestern Scrambled Egg Burritos 170
Smoothie Bowl With Greek Yogurt And Fresh Berries 172
Cherry-Vanilla Baked Oatmeal 174
High-Protein Pancakes 177
Pumpkin Muffins With Walnuts And Zucchini 179
Hard-Boiled Eggs And Avocado On Toast 182
Chapter 3: Vegetarian Dinners 184
Mexican Stuffed Summer Squash...184

Roasted Vegetable Quinoa Salad With Chickpeas 187

Part 1

Introduction

In the past decade, the amount of individuals in the US who have signed up for and gone through with bariatric surgery — specifically the Vertical Sleeve Gastrectomy — have increased by three times. This surgical procedure called the Vertical Sleeve Gastrectomy or "the sleeve" as it has been nicknamed is steadily on the way to being the most frequent of its fellow bariatric cousins. This is a huge deal because it used to be one of the lesser used surgeries compared to the adjustable gastric band and Roux-en-Y gastric bypass, but now it is way out of their league by a lot of miles.

The bariatric procedure is by far the most efficient and lasting way of achieving and maintaining a significant loss of weight, especially when you have tried other methods unsuccessfully. This surgical procedure has proven to be an effective tool for individuals who have dealt with obesity for more years than they can count. It is also a tested and trusted solution for those whose health conditions are way beyond their control.

As you no doubt already know, obesity can greatly affect your quality of life. This is something VSG can help with. It is also recommended for people who would really appreciate a major drop in weight within a fairly short period of time. If you're reading this book, you most likely fit into one of the categories mentioned above or you know someone who does. Either way, if you're opting for a Vertical Sleeve Gastrectomy (VSG), or any of its bariatric cousins, the effects will be lasting and worthwhile.

A major key to effective recovery and success post operation is leaning heavily on your diet. The bariatric diet is very specific and must be followed to the letter. Don't worry, it isn't suffocating or anything because it can totally be adjusted to suit your taste and needs. But! Commitment is key, lovelies. These guidelines and recovery strategies will ensure you achieve maximum physical and mental success. Even more, you will be noticeably healthier than others who choose weight loss strategies that leave them looking sickly and thin.

Type "bariatric surgery diet" into the Google search bar and you'll be hit with over 350,000 results. This much information on a particular topic at just one search can be safely considered information overload, which is why I don't get surprised when people get very confused about meal plans and what to eat after the bariatric procedure.

My interest in VSG diets started after an encounter with my aunt who had undergone the procedure. Assisting her through recovery gave me the opportunity to do a lot of research and meet a lot of other people on the same journey. Then I discovered something: A lot of people who just got sleeved or have plans to get the procedure done for one reason or the other usually have no idea what to eat.

They seemed so eager for nutritional information that are tailored to suit their dietary needs. On that note, I took the time to compile a cookbook for people pre-op and post-op. This cookbook is well armed with enough recipes for the first few weeks post op. If you recently had the VSG procedure done, do not despair! With this book in your armory, you won't ever be worried about what to eat or how to prepare or buy meals you need for proper recovery. I also covered when and how much to eat. You're welcome!

This book is about more than just recipes. This special book contains guidelines for eating post operation from the first day until you're completely transitioned into your normal eating patterns. I'm sure you must know by now that eating doesn't revolve around providing fuel for our bodies. It is much more than that. Eating has a vital emotional aspect as well. Luckily for you, my book covers both the nutritional and emotional aspects of eating especially during this journey. The goal is the initial post op success and of course, long-term success as well.

If you just had your bariatric procedure done, I'd like to say congratulations! You did it, you made it. You made the choice to walk away from whatever diet is in vogue, the most current eating habits, the recent overbearing weight-loss trend and to walk straight into a healthier lifestyle — and you went through with it! You did the right thing by making your decision to lose some pounds.

You know you have jumped one major hurdle, but now you are aware that you will need to get every tool necessary to work on and fit into your new life. I bet you find yo-yo dieting completely exhausting. It's a good thing you have finally taken steps to reach permanent weight loss goals. You deserve this.

You know you deserve to feel lighter than you are used to. You know how deserving you are of more energy than you're used to. You'd like to do the most basic life activities with more ease than you're used to, wouldn't you? More importantly, you should have a healthy weight-loss journey and lifestyle. Breathing should be easier. No one wants to pop medication like it's candy, so be glad you're taking steps to be healthier! You should have a chance to experience all the perks that come with possessing a sound body and mind. This book is the starter pack you need.

First we'll take a good look at the surgery and all there is to know about it, then we'll get into eating guidelines before the recipes start rolling in. Let's go!

Chapter 1: Bariatric Surgeries

We'll start with a definition. If you are reading this out of curiosity, you must be wondering what I have been talking about all throughout the introduction. Bariatric surgery is defined as a medical procedure that alters the levels of hormones in the gut responsible for hunger. It is a procedure that is now more linked to lasting nutritional deficiencies that usually have negative effects on affected individuals.

Most people fall into the pit called malnutrition while on their journey to "permanent weight loss." These risks, in addition to other associated diseases like hypertension, respiratory abnormalities, diabetes mellitus, malignancies, coronary cardiovascular disease and many others, have to be taken into consideration when deciding to go the surgical route to weight loss.

Psychological aspects of living with obesity should also be taken into consideration as it is a very vital factor to consider when choosing to go the surgical route. Living with obesity comes with psychosocial side effects like low self-esteem, reduced quality of life, negative body image, self-hate, and depression. These factors are usually among the list of complaints made by patients who opt for bariatric surgery.

Obesity, according to the CDC statistics, is a chronic illness that has affected about a third of the adults living in the United States of America with a body mass index greater than 40. They also say that another third of adults living in the United States of America are overweight with a body mass index above 30. Dealing with obesity through the surgical route can ensure a permanent and lasting weight-loss plan that is unmatched by countless diets, diet pills, workout routines, hypnosis, meal substitutes, support groups, and behavior adjustments. These other methods might produce initial results, but have not really been able to achieve and maintain long-term success.

Bariatric surgery as a weight-loss method has caused a lot of controversy since it became a thing around the late 1950s. This was due to a lot of failures and complications mid-surgery. However, due to recent developments and major adjustments in the procedure, perioperative complications and failure have reduced by more than 60%. A statistical review conducted in January 2007 by the Agency for Healthcare Research and Quality showed that the total amount of bariatric surgeries conducted from 1998 to 2004 were about ninefold of the number of surgeries conducted before then. The numbers rose from 13,386 to 121,055.

Scientific American released a report that shows the amount spent by the average obese individual in society every single year. The numbers amount to over $7,000, which goes into all the medical treatments and lost productivity. Research conducted at the George Washington University revealed that medical costs for the average overweight person can amount to about $30,000 in a lifetime. Guess what isn't that expensive and is more effective. You guessed it! Bariatric surgery. It remains at the top of the weight-loss chart as the most effective weight loss tool.

Types of Bariatric Surgery

The first bariatric surgical procedures were focused on placing a limit on calorie or nutrient absorption. Kreman and others managed to achieve weight loss by making food go past and avoiding a major portion of the intestines. Over the years, modifications to the initial procedure gave rise to the Roux-en-Y gastroenterostomy, which I'll explain right away.

Roux-en-Y Gastric Bypass

I'll start with a basic description of the procedure:

- It limits the amount of food a person can consume and goes on to affect nutrient absorption.

- It is responsible for a major improvement in blood pressure and blood sugar levels.

- It has been reported to induce 50 to 60% weight loss.

- It causes a dumping syndrome and sometimes, mineral and vitamin deficiencies.

- It has been reported to aid in the decrease in symptoms of type 2 diabetes mellitus.

- It causes constipation and vomiting.

- It can cause lactose intolerance in some patients.

- It can lead to incisional hernia and anemia.

The Roux-en-Y Gastroenterostomy/Gastric Bypass surgery (RYGB) is a medical procedure that involves the major reduction of the size of the stomach to produce a tiny pouch into which food is emptied from the esophagus. During this procedure, the small intestine is sliced through at a specific point underneath the stomach, and then linked to the small pouch.

This creates some kind of bypass through which food goes past most of the stomach and a portion of the small intestine. You know that portion of the small intestine left unused and is still linked to the old stomach? That portion is put in a loop around the used portion of the small intestine and connected to it to create a "Y" shape. All this rewiring is to make room for the drainage of gastric juices.

You must be wondering how one can lose weight through this process. Well, weight loss through this procedure will occur from the new limits placed on food consumption and the new changes that will occur in the hormonal and neuronal pathways as a result of all the cutting and connecting that was done. The combination of these will ensure weight loss. Most of the studies conducted on the gastric bypass procedures have reported that a lot of people who have rapid weight loss from this surgery are at a great risk of developing gallstones and therefore might have to have their gallbladder removed during the procedure to eliminate those risks completely.

Reports have shown no major difference in the survival rates of at about a month and a year between obese patients who opt for a gastric bypass surgery and others who chose against it. An omega loop gastric bypass which is also called a mini-gastric bypass or single anastomosis gastric bypass has been on the rise all through Asia and in some European countries. Studies conducted on the procedure have claimed it to be a quick, effective and safe bariatric procedure that ensures the expected weight loss in comparison to the RYGB.

Vertical Sleeve Gastrectomy

I'll start with a basic description of the procedure:

- Like the RYGB, it limits the amount of food consumed by a person and the reduction of the hormones responsible for hunger.

- It cannot be changed to a gastric bypass.

- It involves a vertical division of the stomach and a permanent removal of about 70 to 80% of the stomach

- There is no rerouting of intestines involved.

- It can cause acid reflux

- It is a permanent procedure.

- It has been reported to induce about 50 to 60% weight loss

Vertical Sleeve Gastrectomy or VSG is quickly becoming the surgery of choice for a lot of patients and surgeons due to how easy the procedure is, as well as the complete bypass of bowel rearrangement. That said, I should point out it is likely to come with lifelong complications. This surgery came to be in 1988 and was called a Biliopancreatic Diversion with Duodenal Switch (BPD-DS).

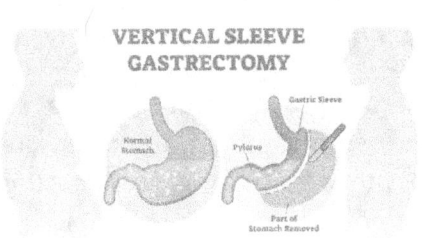

Weight loss happens when food portions are limited and the amount of nutrients absorbed is also limited. This kind of bariatric procedure has proven to be better than other procedures when it comes to weight loss for both long-term and short-term. However, a lot of patients and surgeons have left this procedure behind despite the obvious results for a more improved version — the VSG — as well as the Roux-en-Y gastroenterostomy.

Curious about what happens during the VSG procedure? Here, about 70 to 80% of the stomach is removed along the greater curvature.

Some important parts of the stomach like the pylorus are left intact. When you eat, the bolus is ground per usual, and sent into the duodenal loop, the first stop on its journey to digestion and absorption. After the VSG procedure, your stomach should look like a long slim banana. The size of this banana depends on your surgeon. Increased complications of this surgery includes Gastroesophageal Reflux Disease (GERD). This problem is most associated with patients who get a much smaller sleeve than usual. A typical stomach can contain roughly 1500ml, but this procedure ensures reduction to about 90ml to 200ml.

As you must have realized, a smaller stomach automatically equals smaller food intake and quick satiety (you get full faster than you're used to). Despite all this, to lose weight and maintain results, certain lifestyle changes have to take effect or else changes in hormones that tell your brain when you've had enough food can affect your success negatively.

Some research has proven that filling a sleeve with saline increases the pressure to about 43mmHg, unlike the 34mmHg that is shown with a full stomach. The surgery pretty much lessens the ability of the stomach to expand very much, thereby inducing early satiety and decreasing food consumption.

Another thing to know is that when you undergo VSG, a lot of cells responsible for the production of ghrelin — also called the hunger hormone — are lost in the process. This is another major aspect of appetite control in this procedure. Normally, when ghrelin is released in your body, appetite and the growth hormone are stimulated so you feel hunger.

It is also an important weight regulator as it determines when you should eat. Studies have shown that the levels Of ghrelin become greatly reduced and stay reduced for up to 6 months after the surgery. This is important for the weight loss that needs to happen post op.

Laparoscopic Sleeve Gastrectomy or LSG is also on the rise, according to studies on the subject. LSG ensures lower rates of morbidity, lesser operative time, reduced rate of wound infections, and fewer occurrences of blood loss. Sleeve gastrectomy is usually accompanied by folate and vitamin D deficiencies which occur before and after the procedure. However fewer deficiencies have been reported from VSG than RYGB.

Stomach Intestinal Pylorus Sparing Surgery

Here is a basic description of the procedure:

- This procedure ensures a slightly bigger sleeve than the others.

- Instead of being attached to the distal ileum, it is connected to the mid small intestine.

- It results in ghrelin suppression.

- Less of the bowel is lost in this procedure for the prevention of bowel disorders.

- It's just like Vertical Sleeve Gastrectomy, which involves shortening the intestines.

Stomach Intestinal Pylorus Sparing Surgery (SIPS) is an improved version of the duodenal switch surgery that works to reduce health issues related to the bowel like diarrhea. It also works to induce weight loss through ghrelin reduction. This procedure doesn't get rid of the pyloric valve just like the Vertical Sleeve Gastrectomy, and it also does not bypass a major portion of the small intestine like the RYGB.

Also, the absence of a roux limb and distal anastomosis is believed to greatly lessen the risk of intestinal obstruction in the long-term, and also decrease gastrointestinal symptoms. The risk of bile reflux gastritis hasn't been reported to increase because of the attachment is located after the stomach valve. This surgery is usually recommended for patients who have undergone VSG but regained weight or didn't lose as much weight as they would've liked.

Adjustable Gastric Banding

Here's what happens with this procedure:

- Just like other bariatric surgeries, it limits food consumption.

- It is a less invasive procedure than the rest and this leads to quicker recovery.

- The procedure is not irreversible.

- It leads to weight loss, but moderately.

- Any foreign object in the body will be easily removed.

- This surgery has a high rate of reoperation because there are risks of erosion or bandage slippage.

Adjustable Gastric Banding (AGB), which is also called LAP-BAND, is belt that is filled with fluid which is looped around the stomach to form an upper pouch into which food goes straight from the esophagus and then drains through the lower pouch and into the intestines.

I'm going to tell you something really cool about this belt: It has a tiny tube that the surgeon connects to a port just underneath the stomach. So, you must wonder what a straight tube from the belt to the stomach is used for. Well, with this tube, the surgeon can adjust the amount of fluid in the belt to loosen or tighten it. The tightness of the belt regulates the flow of food between the upper and lower pouches of the stomach. How easily food moves from point A to point B depends on how tight the belt is.

Sometime in 2011, people with a body mass index of 30 or more instead of the usual minimum of 35 were now allowed to apply for bariatric surgeries. This development was voted in by an advisory panel in the Food and Drug Administration. This is because they have probably tried other weight loss methods like workout routines, extreme diet and appetite suppression drugs. These methods must have failed them and led them to look into bariatric procedures.

LAP-BAND is a strictly restrictive procedure that is used to regulate food consumption. The mortality rate for this surgery is very low and it ensures weight loss, too, but gradually. This procedure is usually recommended for patients with regular workout routines and strict diet choices. Adjustments on the belt can be done every 5 to 7 weeks at the hospital. This is most important especially in cases of pregnancy.

This method ensures weight loss which is not necessarily permanent, because despite the regulation of food intake, some patients can regain a bit or all of the weight by bingeing on soft foods like ice cream or smoothies with high carbs content and other soft foods rich in fat. This happens because there was no work done to modify absorption rate. Therefore, proper diet and discipline is very important for long term success.

Vitamins and other nutritional supplements will be recommended by your physician. You'll have to take these as long as it is needed to ensure your body gets the necessary vitamins, trace minerals, proteins, and calcium it needs to function.

A major complication in this procedure is the gastric band slippage. This challenge is so major that it can cause pain, dysphagia, and affect weight loss. When the band slips, the patient will need to get revision surgery. Band slippage is most associated with poor diet compliance post-op, this means if you don't eat what you have been told to, how you have been told to, and when you have been told to, you risk your tummy belt slipping off.

What You Gain From All This

Studies have shown a great improvement with RYGB in mitochondrial disorders found in adipose tissue which results in Type 2 diabetes mellitus. However, if you opt for a weight loss surgery that isn't as aggressive, you may not get the same results. Other studies have shown reduced glycemic control and a lack of improvement in that area over time following AGB.

However, bariatric surgeries still get top billing when it comes to lasting weight loss as opposed to rigorous exercising and dieting. The first year post-op is usually all roses and rainbows because of the new habits, new body, improved esteem, new diet choices, and so on. However, a lot of patients start to relapse really quickly.

The former president of the American Society for Metabolic and Bariatric Surgery, Dr John Morton, who also happens to be the head of bariatric surgery at Stanford University School of Medicine in California, stated that bariatric patients who end up putting on the lost pounds post-op can still enjoy certain health benefits from the procedure. The medical director of the University of Virginia, the department of surgery in Charlottesville, Virginia, Peter T. Hallowell and a few of his colleagues took time to study bariatric surgeries in about 401 patients. Their reports showed clear success post-op in obese and overweight patients who chose to undergo a gastrectomy, compared to those who decided against it.

The benefits of this procedure can also be enjoyed by teens who have major difficulty losing weight despite engaging in more physical activities and making sure to eat healthy foods. Adolescents at about 16 years old with a BMI of 40 and above can be put under consideration for a surgical solution to prevent further challenges that come with obesity. Also, this kind of surgery works to regulate the brain's reward system, curbing the sweet tooth so adolescent patients may benefit more from this route than other weight loss programs.

What is Gastric Sleeve Surgery?

Now you know what a bariatric procedure entails and the various ones currently on the market, so let's turn our attention to the Gastric Sleeve Surgery. This is one of the bariatric surgeries I mentioned above. It can also be called a Vertical Sleeve Gastrectomy (VSG) or a Sleeve Gastrectomy. This special surgery limits the amount of food you can eat so you lose weight much easier than you would if you keep eating as much as you'd like. Fun fact: You can actually lose about 50lbs - 90lbs through this procedure.

It all starts as a laparoscopic surgery with tiny cuts or incisions on the upper stomach before more than half of the left portion of the stomach is taken out. Whatever is left of your stomach should look like a narrow tube which people call the "sleeve." Food enters through your mouth, down your esophagus, into your sleeve and into your small intestines just like before but this time, your stomach is much tinier. Your small intestine will be left alone, unharmed during the surgery and after, you'll feel full after just a small pack of chips. Intriguing huh?

Why Should You Opt For a Gastric Sleeve Surgery?

This procedure is mostly recommended for treatment of morbid obesity. If you have dabbled in other traditional weight loss therapies and failed or not had any lasting success, this procedure is what you need. Your physician is likely to recommend a gastric sleeve surgery if you are morbidly obese with a BMI of 40 and above. Your physician may also recommend this surgery if your body mass index is somewhere around 35 and 40 and you're also dealing with health issues like diabetes mellitus, high blood pressure, coronary problems and sleep apnea.

What Are The Risks of Gastric Sleeve Surgery?

Possible side effects of getting sleeved include but are not limited to infection, thrombosis (blood clots) in the legs, and bleeding. Allergies to general anesthesia are also very possible and dangerous as they can cause breathing problems, hives, swollen eyes, and other allergic reactions.

In the long term, you might have issues with the absorption of some nutrients or you may end up developing a narrowing in the sleeve. Some patients have reported heartburn post-op. My aunt, for example, experienced acid reflux for a few days after the surgery. If you have already been experiencing acid reflux before the procedure no matter how moderate, getting sleeved could worsen that. So, it is advisable to opt for a gastric bypass procedure. With that, you can say bye to heartburn and acid reflux forever. You should discuss with your physician first because you might have other health related risks that might affect the procedure during and post-op.

How Do I Get Ready for Gastric Sleeve Surgery?

First of all, you'll have to consult with your healthcare professional, because only they can determine if getting sleeved is a good idea for you. Bariatric surgery isn't usually recommended for individuals who are into drug or alcohol abuse. It isn't advised for people who have difficulty committing to long-term diet changes and workout routines.

Weeks before the surgery takes place, your physician may recommend you join a bariatric surgery preparation program. This will give you the support and education you need while preparing for the journey pre-op and post-op. You will be given nutritional counseling, which is very important for this procedure. You might also get a psych-eval just to be sure you are ready for the next chapter of your life. You'll undergo a number of tests and physical examinations. Blood tests, too. So if you're a tiny bit afraid of needles, you'll need to be brave for this one.

You might also do a bit of imaging so the pros can see what they'll be working with and prepare for everything. If you're a smoker, you'll be asked to stop several months before the procedure date. Your physician might even ask that you shed a few pounds before the surgery because this will ensure that your liver gets small enough for the procedure. A tinier liver means a safer surgery in this case. If you take blood thinners like ibuprofen or aspirin, you will be asked to stop a few days before your surgery. Another given is that you will need to stay away from any food and drinks after midnight on the day before your procedure.

What Happens During Gastric Sleeve Surgery

You will be given a general anesthetic for the procedure. This means you will be in la-la land throughout the action. Trust me when I say you won't be missing much. Your physician will perform laparoscopy, which is basically poking around in your abdomen with a fancy torchlight to see what's in it.

How this happens is the physician will make some incisions on the upper part of your abdomen, then insert the laparoscope (fancy torchlight) and the necessary tools for your procedure into these small cuts. When that is all set up, the person in charge of anesthesia (the anesthesiologist) will place a sizing tube into your mouth and slide it down your esophagus into your stomach.

Once the sizing tube is in your stomach, a laparoscopic stapler will be used to separate your stomach into the portion that will be removed and the one that won't. This will leave you with a narrowed stomach. Your very own sleeve. The portion of your stomach that should be removed will be cut off and brought out of the body through one of the tiny incisions I mentioned earlier. Once all this is done and you are left with your sleeve, the surgeon will check for any leakage in the sleeve using an upper endoscopy or a dye test.

What Happens After Gastric Sleeve Surgery?

You will likely be discharged from the hospital the next day. You will be told to stay on a strictly liquid diet for a week or two post-op. Your healthcare professional will provide you with a diet plan for proper recovery over the coming weeks. The process is typically liquid foods, to purees, then soft foods, before bouncing back to regular meals. As expected, each meal portion will be very small. For your own sake, eat as slowly as possible and chew on each bite properly. Take your time with this transition. Moving too quickly to regular food can affect your healing process, so take it slow. Regular food during this time can cause you pain and nausea.

When your stomach does heal, you know by now that you need to change your eating habits. Your meal portions will be much smaller to fit the new size of your stomach. One of the major diet challenges patients have after this procedure is mineral and vitamin absorption. They no longer get as much as they used to through meals, because they eat less food now, which automatically means less nutrients. Your medical team should recommend certain supplements for you post-op, like a daily multivitamin, plus some calcium and vitamin D supplements. Depending on your progress, you might need extra nutrients like iron and vitamin B-12. All these will be determined by your healthcare professional.

Regular checkups and blood tests in the next few months following your surgery are very important because you will need to make sure you're not suffering any vitamin deficiencies, low blood iron, low calcium, or high glucose levels. If you experience heartburn post-op, you may have to get medications that reduce stomach acid levels.

When you lose weight post-op, it is very possible to pack those pounds back on in no time. To ensure this doesn't happen, you have to strictly follow a healthy diet plan and engage in regular workouts. Keep in mind that despite this being a permanent procedure, it is possible for the sleeve to dilate over a period of time and a bigger sleeve equals bigger meal portions, so if you eat as much as your wider sleeve lets you, you'll start to pack on the pounds and everything you've been through would have been for nothing. You should consider becoming a part of a bariatric support group to assist you in better fitting into your new life and habits.

Why Get Sleeved?

Getting a Vertical Sleeve Gastrectomy is a very important and clearly life changing decision. This particular surgery has some advantages over other bariatric surgeries. Why get sleeved? I'll tell you!

You get your own inbuilt portion control system: With your current knowledge of the procedure, you know that more than half of your stomach will be removed. With just 15 to 20 percent of your abdomen remaining after the procedure, the amount of food you can eat at a go will be limited by a lot. This doesn't mean you won't enjoy meals anymore. You'll still enjoy a gazillion dishes, starting with the really soft foods while you and your sleeve work your way up to meals of a more solid consistency. The fact remains that your stomach will give you a heads up when it's full so you can stop eating.

Your hunger signals take a nosedive: The removal of a large portion of your stomach brings with it a drop in ghrelin production. Less ghrelin equals less feelings of "I want to eat" and feeling less of that will definitely make you eat less.

You shed up to more than half your initial body weight: Excess body weight is the extra weight besides that which is appropriate for your height. Healthy weight isn't really determined by how much flesh is on a person's bones because that amount might be perfect for their height. Studies conducted by the American Society for Metabolic and Bariatric Surgery have shown that obese patients who have undergone the sleeve gastrectomy usually lose about 55 percent of their initial body weight, and are able to maintain this loss for about 5 years or longer post-op. If your excess body weight is about 150 pounds — that is minus your ideal body weight, — this means that you'll shed at least 80 pounds or more and maintain this weight loss.

You will be able to appreciate your sweet tooth when it comes to the dumping syndrome: A lot of people, including myself, have a difficult time with the idea of giving up all the sweet goodies forever after undergoing any weight loss surgery. I can't imagine a life without being able to taste a birthday cake or candy for the rest of my life. That said, I bet you're wondering what dumping syndrome is. It is a special condition that can affect people who have undergone gastric bypass surgery. What happens is when they eat a lot of carbs at once or foods with high sugar content at a go, they start to feel lightheaded, dizzy, and shaky. All these happen within a few minutes after consumption. Think of a sugar rush, but in a really bad way. Sometimes, they might experience stomach aches, diarrhea, elevated heartrate and other very uncomfortable symptoms. I'm not saying it is completely impossible to experience dumping syndrome after getting sleeved, but it is very rare. If and when it does occur, it doesn't feel as terrible as it would've been if you opted for a gastric bypass because in VSG, your intestines will be completely left alone.

You will spend less time on the operating table: All surgeries come with risks and potential complications, but the ones that involve putting a person under a general anesthesia pose an even greater risk. These risks become worse if the amount of time needed to complete the surgery is major. The longer a person stays under, the greater the risks. The VSG, despite taking longer than the adjustable band procedure, is a much quicker and easier surgery than the BPD-DS and gastric bypass.

Chapter 2: A New You

It's completely normal to want to be part of a society, a clan, a group or a club. Good thing is, there's a VSG club and you just became a member! This club is strictly for people who have plans to get sleeved and people who have already been sleeved. Being there and taking care of my aunt, I can say that I understand the difficulties people have to go through way before and in the days leading up to the surgery date. When you make the choice to get this done and to turn your life around, and when you share this awesome news with anyone you can, you will get all kinds of responses.

Some will be supportive. Others, not so much. They might tell you that you seem to be searching for an easy route out of your problem or that surgery is risky and drastic. What you have to do is trash these comments and put one truth on repeat: You are a strong person. This club, no matter how unofficial it is, is filled with the strength of a thousand survivors; people who decided to take a stand in their life and turn everything around for the better with the help of a medical professional. You are strong. You are brave. Congratulations on your new life!

Begin Again With Food

When choosing to undergo the Vertical Sleeve Gastrectomy, you will definitely have a full team of healthcare professionals, including a surgeon, a psychologist, and a qualified dietitian, among others. It will be their job to assist you in properly understanding the process and how to properly prepare for it mentally, nutritionally, and of course, physically.

However, after the procedure, although you will still have your supportive healthcare professional, your progress will really depend on your ability to start over with food. This is a brand-new chapter of your life, and while you might have instructions, dos and don'ts from your physician, you will need to do a lot of self-education on the matter of nutrition.

You are solely in charge of your progress and success. This self-management can make things a little difficult for you, but don't be afraid. I will go over some of the difficulties people experience post-op and how to manage them like a pro.

Embracing Eating Without Fear

Undergoing bariatric surgery means you will have to learn to eat from scratch. You will begin with liquids and slowly work your way up to a balanced diet made up of all the things you used to eat before — but with a healthy twist. It is completely understandable to be afraid of food because of the uncertainty that comes with it. It's okay to be afraid of not knowing what to eat and what to avoid. Also, it is normal to be afraid of going back to your bad eating habits and messing up all your progress. A way to conquer this fear is to embrace your new life without fear.

During this transitional stage, you should set your mind on things you can eat and not the things you can't. You should stick to the simple rules of the bariatric diet and focus on the foods you know you can have or at least try. This is not going to be an easy journey.

It might take a lot of time for you to get acquainted with the dos and don'ts of your new lifestyle, so you have to cut yourself some slack, give yourself some patience, and have faith in yourself. Don't be quick to do food experiments because your stomach isn't ready for that yet. If you follow the diet rules to the letter, you reduce your chances of getting sick to 0.3%. You just have to follow the rules and pay attention to your body.

Mindful Eating

During this period, you will need to practice a bit of mindfulness. You need to be in tune with your body and stop eating the minute your body tells you it's done. Listen to your body's natural signs and do everything you can to stop yourself from taking another bite after your body tells you it can't take anymore, because it literally can't. You might be used to eating more than that, but that was when you had a regular sized stomach. Now your stomach is way less than regular sized, so it's only logical to eat much less. You don't have to be afraid. Your body will let you know when it has had enough.

Decide, Commit, and You'll Succeed

You need to develop a strong commitment to yourself. This is not going to be like those countless times you went on a diet and quit. This is unlike anything you've done before. This time, your body has been altered and you have to act accordingly. The fear of going back to the old you who never finished whatever they started will definitely hit and it might hit hard. However, you need to keep in mind that this time is and will be different. Your banana tummy gives you a head start which none of the other diets did. This isn't just a weight loss diet; it is a weight loss lifestyle. A lasting, and hopefully permanent weight loss lifestyle.

Support Systems Matter

You will need to recognize and accept the importance of support in this situation. You should have some faith in your healthcare professional, as they really have your best interests at heart. You should also rely on family and maybe a few friends or even colleagues. Anyone you trust is a shoulder to lean on during this stage and I assure you, you will need that shoulder.

You should learn to open up to the ones you trust whenever you feel scared. They care for you and will encourage you. You might think you don't really have a shoulder to lean on, but maybe it's just because you haven't really looked. You should look and look hard. There is someone or even a bunch of someone's who will be there for.

For some, it might be a bariatric support group, a therapist, a friend, a pastor, or even a health coach. Whoever it is, try to really connect with them because they're the ones who will get you through the rough patches that will come. A life of fear is mentally and physically crippling. You need to reassure yourself and be full of confidence in your own strength.

Managing Urges

Everyone has urges. Everyone. Be it a second round of dessert or an impulsive purchase at the supermarket. It can also be a wasted day with missed workouts and one less Netflix episode to watch. Life somehow finds creative ways to make us submit to impulse and eventually fall off your healthy wagon. Manage the urges that come post-op comes in two ways:

- **Mindful behavior:** A certain awareness of your actions, thoughts, and feelings will help you better deal with your urges.

Living in the present can really help suppress these strong impulses because then you will be in control, not on autopilot.

- **Resisting cravings:** Giving in to a craving can mean opening a door that has been long shut or flipping a switch. This can be turning into the person you thought you threw in the trash. Having one chip can turn into the whole bag. A simple glass of wine can slowly become half a bottle. A lot of bariatric patients are at risk of falling into binge eating each time they give into an impulse, no matter how tiny.

Instead, be mindful and be in tune with your body and its needs. Sometimes, your body might tell you it needs that ice cream or candy, but instead of just giving in, ask again to be sure so you don't lose all you've gained for one tiny piece of candy.

Demonstrating Self-Compassion

I don't know if anyone has ever told you this, but the way you feel about yourself and treat yourself after bad and good behavior has a direct effect on your happiness. This can also affect your commitment and ability to be dedicated to the long-term changes that come with surgery. Self-compassion can be split into three basic things: Mindfulness, humanity, and self-kindness.

If you think for one second that it is possible to have a flawless recovery with zero mistakes and zero slip ups, then you are setting yourself up for a whole different kind of disappointment. Everyone makes mistakes post-op. The difference is how you react to yours. Do you react with self-criticism or self-compassion? This is part of the determinants of our resilience after a moment of relapse. Nobody is perfect. All we can do is accept our imperfections and reward our good qualities.

If you unfairly criticize yourself every time you make a mistake, you only work to move yourself farther down the progress ladder. To avoid self-denigration, you should understand that you will have a few bad days. When you do, you should accept that your mind might just need a break. Try moving past your mistakes without dwelling too much on how you could've done things differently. It is all part of the journey.

Appreciating Natural Sweetness

Unfortunately, our world is one where the threshold for sweet just keeps increasing. Sweet beverages are getting even sweeter, and desserts are sugarier than before. Letting go of our love for added sugars can be extremely difficult for people on a weight-loss journey because honestly, sugar is addictive. Every time we eat sugary foods, the pleasure centers of our brain lights up, and makes you want to go back and get some more, because we all like our pleasure centers being lit up as often as possible.

The downside is the calories start to pile up. The pounds start showing. This is very bad... and I don't even mean aesthetically. A lot of health complications come with obesity as you must already know. If sugar addiction is a problem you are dealing with, a VSG gives you a once in a lifetime opportunity to hit reset. Your eating patterns get a complete makeover that's necessary if you're going to kick old habits out of your life.

What you should do when you get this second chance is learn to appreciate natural sweetness. This will satisfy your sweet tooth and help keep that banging waistline. Grains like quinoa and barley have a natural sweetness to them, and are still packed with a lot of nutrients. If you must have something obviously sweet, instead of punishing your body with sugary beverages and desserts, why don't you just have a bowl of mixed berries or a glass of freshly squeezed orange juice? If you have a chocolate craving, you can satisfy that by using 100% cocoa powder when making protein shakes instead of the calorie-packed chocolate candies that have overrun the market. You have a second chance. Do things differently!

Dealing With Weight Loss Expectations

The concept of weight-loss is not an exact science. Even weight loss researchers know that in controlled weight loss studies, variations on just how much weight a person can lose will occur. It is pretty annoying when you invest your all time and then some into something, only to get less than half of the expected results. Managing your weight loss expectations is key during this period.

To do this, you have to stop putting unnecessary pressure on yourself. You need to accept that the timeline you set for yourself might be a little too unrealistic if you think about it. You need to understand your body and give it time. Come to terms with the fact that people lose weight at different paces. Some will definitely shed the pounds faster than you will.

This does not mean there is anything wrong with you. There are a lot of factors that come into consideration when thinking about weight loss. A number of these factors are beyond your control. I bet you didn't know that sleep is one of these factors. Other factors include initial body weight, age, stress, height, muscle mass, gender, and so on.

Do your best but be patient with yourself. Give yourself more time than you currently are and try not to compare your journey to anyone else's. It is your journey and not theirs.

Enjoying Food Again

Eating right after surgery can be very uncomfortable especially in the few days following the procedure when you have to consume a lot of liquids. During this stage, if you find yourself hating food or imagining how to never eat again, it's fine. It's all a part of the process. At first, eating will feel like washing the steps or doing homework. The questions will start rolling in: *Will I ever want to eat the foods I loved before surgery? Is it possible for me to ever look forward to meals again?*

To answer your questions, yes you will. I need you to understand that a lot of changes will happen in your body right after surgery. Physical and hormonal changes will take place, all trying to get you to eat less. So don't beat yourself up if you cooperate. A bulk of the initial weight loss can be attributed to these changes. Give yourself time. Give your body time.

As your healing process progresses, you will find yourself wanting to eat other things, and have a bit more than before. You will find your tolerance has greatly increased. I don't mean to scare you, but there's a good chance you won't crave ice cream and pizza like you used to. I have seen it happen time and time again.

This is because with the transition into this special diet packed with healthy meal options, you will notice your cravings leaving the high-calorie section and leaning towards the healthy section. The moment you experience this, know that you can start experimenting with food.

You can jazz up old recipes of food you used to like to make it suit your current lifestyle. That being said, food is necessary for life. We all need it to function. Your appetite will improve with time, but you have to be patient with yourself.

The Sweet Stuff

This procedure has a lot of differences from the BPD/DS or gastric bypass. This means VSG patients don't experience some of the complications those other patients have, like the dumping syndrome. This automatically means that sweets and desserts in healthy portions are not totally off the table post-op. After the surgery, you may have feelings of being left out. You may not feel normal again. All that is temporary. Soon, you will be back to enjoying these things in moderation!

Eating at restaurants, parties, or even family gatherings can be a real bother if you have to always make people understand why you're staying away from dessert. Getting sleeved provides a little bit of flexibility compared to other bariatric procedures, but never in the beginning. The good thing is, you'll be giving fewer explanations at some point. However, you still have to be mindful and ensure you don't overindulge.

How Not to Overindulge

- Try not to have tempting desserts in your house.
- When you do indulge, lean more on portion-controlled tiny individual servings instead of a buffet with the big bag.
- Whatever you do, candies shouldn't be kept at your desk.

Studies have proven that sitting down with an entire bag of chips means you're likely to eat much more than you would have done if you were given a portion-controlled serving, or a smaller bite on a plate. Always do it the portion-controlled way. A single serving is the best way to go.

Even if you go for a second serving, you will still end up having less than normal which is really good. My point is, if you want sweets, then they don't have to completely be erased from the equation. You'll just have to do it the sleeved way now.

Chapter 3: Eating Guidelines For Pre-Op And Post-Op

Meal Planning

A diet plan should become a major part of your new, exciting life, post VSG. Think of it like brushing your hair every morning or even dressing up every morning before you leave the house. Making a list of meal options for the week does not have to entail writing down every last ingredient. It simply means that you're not entirely clueless about what to eat throughout the week. It means making a mental note of what ingredients are available or easy to obtain and the meal prep you're able to make in preparation for days when you're unable to prepare a meal from scratch.

Meal planning is more important than most people realize in the first few months after the surgery to ensure you get the amount of protein you need. You should make sure your meal plan is based on foods with enough protein, then slowly progress into incorporating vegetables and fruits into the plan. Grains and other regular foods will come in last.

Meal prep allows you to plan your meals way beforehand, so you know you have something healthy handy, in case you need a quick fix. It takes that day-to-day stress out of the picture. Also, meal prep saves you time. The longer it takes to prepare a meal, the hungrier you get. We don't want you ravenous, do we?

With meal plans and meal preps, you reduce the chances of you ever going to grab a quick, probably unhealthy fix at a fast food joint. It's better if you make time to prepare a meal that you can eat more than twice. Freeze whatever leftovers you have and microwave them later. Place food portions into disposable containers and place them in the freezer to make your own frozen meal. Make a list of the things you have in your fridge, when you prepared it, and where exactly you put it so you won't get confused or lost when searching for it.

Meals that have a sauce happen to freeze really well and remain moist when microwaved. I'll tell you a trick: Each time you make a frozen dinner, you give the flavors a chance to really come together. This is why leftovers almost always taste better than freshly prepared meals.

The first few months after the surgery isn't going to be all sunshine and rainbows. It will be difficult and might take you a while to adjust to, especially when it comes to diet. This is why I took some time to prepare a meal plan to help you through the first eight weeks after the procedure. I put some easy and super tasty recipes in later chapters, but first we'll go over the basics.

VSG Nutritional Know-How

Getting a Vertical Sleeve Gastrectomy is usually a last resort for most people because they must have tried other traditional weight loss methods and failed. This is why I'm sure you must have background knowledge on popular weight-loss diets. I bet you know a bit about nutritional benefits and certain restrictions that come with weight loss diets like the Mediterranean diet, anti-inflammatory diet, Weight Watchers diet, Atkins diet, and others. The good news is that having some background knowledge about diets and their rules will provide a good foundation for your diet plan and life after surgery.

Anybody who says you need to be an expert in nutrition probably knows less than you do on the topic, because you definitely don't need a degree in nutrition to be able to comprehend and follow the bariatric diet plan. First of all, we'll take a look at the basic rules for formulating a proper bariatric meal plan. Each diet has principles and this one is no different. It is pretty straightforward, if you ask me, and more for your benefit as you'll soon see.

Liquids: Making sure you're properly hydrated after any surgical procedure is a very important rule and even more so for this procedure. Taking an adequate amount of liquids will give you a different kind of energy boost. More than that, it will also greatly assist you in losing weight.

Another thing is that dehydration is one of the most common problems that people experience after surgery. It is also one of the most easily avoidable complications. At first, it might seem like quite a feat because you shouldn't drink anything with meals or drink within 30 minutes of eating only. However, always keep a beverage handy or make sure you can easily purchase one wherever you might be.

Instead of worrying about how you can take in large amounts of water, focus on drinking a little at a time. Make sure you take small amounts of water or any appropriate liquid throughout the day to avoid drowning in thirst and having to drink large amounts of water later. Besides, your tummy is now less than half its original size so you can't even take in large amounts of anything even if you wanted to. To avoid getting frustrated, just take it slow.

What you can drink: Soy milk, water, protein shakes, milk, decaf coffee or tea with zero sugar and zero cream, noncarbonated beverages, sugar-free beverages, which can be substituted with beverages that contain natural sweeteners like stevia.

Amount per day: You should be looking at consuming 64 ounces to a 100 ounces for the first few weeks, before increasing the volume little by little over time.

What you should avoid: Juices, sugar sweetened beverages, caffeinated beverages like energy drinks, soda, tea, and others, alcohol, sports drinks, carbonated water, lemonade, and sweetened tea.

Protein: Protein is everything. It is about the most important macronutrient you will need after the surgery. Each time your body is under maintenance or is working on a new structure within you, it requires protein. No protein, no construction. This is why protein consumption is very important when starting a low calorie diet.

Consuming adequate amounts of protein will leave you feeling full of energy, help with weight loss, and preserve muscle. Another plus is that the satiety you feel when you eat enough food will be doubled. Basically, you will feel full for longer because the digestion of protein takes an even longer time than carbs. Even better, protein has fewer calories than fat and carbs.

During the first few weeks after the surgery, it may seem like all you ever have are water and foods rich in protein. As you get more comfortable with your new life and heal nicely, you will gradually start incorporating other nutrients into your diet plan. This book is filled with various recipe options for you and your recovery. You will find a variety of protein rich foods for the long term so you don't get bored with meals. Having a slice of protein at every meal is not only essential for weight loss and bodybuilding, it is also a requirement for maintaining weight loss in the long haul.

What you can eat: Eggs, poultry like skinless turkey, ground chicken breast, chicken, turkey sausage, lean nitrate-free chicken, and turkey breast; all kinds of seafood; low-fat or nonfat dairy products like 1% nonfat cottage cheese, low fat Greek yogurt, and others; if not a vegetarian, you can have lean beef like loin, lean or supreme lean ground beef, round roast, steak, or sirloin, no less than three months after surgery. You can also have lean pork, tenderloin, ham with all the visible fat taken out, and top loin chop if you are not a vegetarian. This should be around three months after the surgery. Protein sources for vegetarians include nuts, seeds, beans, and lentils.

Amount per day: You should consume around 60 grams to 100 grams of protein. However, speak to your healthcare professional so they can decide the most specific recommendation for your body weight and post-op meal stage.

What you should avoid: High-fat dairy products like whole milk and cream; high-fat beef and pork like bologna, pork sausage, salami, bacon, ground beef, and pork ribs; any poultry with the skin on.

Carbohydrates: Carbs are your best bet when sourcing energy for your entire body and brain. Carbohydrates are an important nutrient needed for a lot of metabolic actions. In the first few weeks post-op, you will be on a strictly no-carb diet. Your body will be just fine running on energy gotten from protein and fat because glucose isn't the only juice your body can take, unlike what you were told. There are two varieties of carbohydrates: Simple carbohydrates, and complex carbohydrates.

Simple carbs are the kind easily digested by the body and quickly converted to glucose in the blood. This super-fast breakdown causes us to get that "sugar rush" we all know too well. It gives us a quick high and an equally quick crash. Simple carbs examples are candies, juice drinks, anything prepared with white refined flour, soda and a lot of processed foods.

Complex carbs are the slow and steady lot. The body takes time to digest them. It's a slow process and doesn't give the famous sugar rush. Complex carbs are rich in vitamins, fiber, and mineral content. They are made up of fruits, 100% whole grain, vegetables, and so on. The goal is to have more complex carbs and less simple carbs.

What you can eat: Vegetables, oatmeal, sweet potatoes or white potatoes with the skin, fresh fruits, wild or brown rice, 100% whole wheat pasta— if your body can tolerate it, 100% whole-grain bread. Toasted bread is easier to tolerate than fresh bread. You can also have barley, ancient grains like farrow, quinoa, millet, spelt, and so on.

Amount per day: You should focus on consuming little to no carbs throughout the first year post-op. For the long term, 35 % of your calorie content should come from carbs.

What you should avoid: Avoid all white refined grain products like white pasta, crackers, white bread; cakes; cookies; pastries; chips; candies; soda; all kinds of juice including natural fruit juice.

Fats: One major importance of dietary fats is the absorption of the essential fat-soluble vitamins (A, D, E and K). Also, there are certain important fatty acids that your body is incapable of synthesizing on its own, so you need to eat them as food instead. For example, omega-3 and omega-6. Among all the macronutrients known to man, fats have the most amount of calories at 9kcal per gram.

Because of the calorie density, we must take extra care when measuring portions, even when it comes to healthy fats. One has to be extra careful with any processed food that claims to be fat-free or low-fat, because they might be fat-free, but what they lack in fats, they have in excess sugar or excess sodium to boost the food's flavor.

When consuming dairy products, especially yogurt, cottage cheese, and milk, it is advisable to eat nonfat or low-fat versions to cut back on calories and unhealthy saturated fats. These versions should make up the bulk of your fat choices.

Important note: 1% milk or nonfat milk does not contain less minerals or minerals than whole milk. The protein content is almost identical too. Always opt for full fat foods like nuts, avocados, fatty fish, vegetable oils and olives. Your heart will love you even more!

What you can eat: Chia seeds, shellfish, avocado, flaxseed, fatty fish like mackerel, tuna and salmon, almonds, nut butters with no additives, walnuts, extra-virgin olive oil, peanuts, and other seafood,

Amount per day: This should be consumed in very limited amounts in the first few weeks post-op. Over the long haul, this nutrient shouldn't make up even 30% of your calorie content per meal. Stick to healthy versions as much as you can and if you must indulge in the unhealthy kind, it should always be less than 7%.

What you should limit: Butter, full fat dairy, tropical oils like coconut and palm oils, miscellaneous vegetable oils.

What you should avoid: Animal fats like the ones gotten from lard and meat; stick margarines that contain trans fats; fried foods; any foods with high saturated fat content.

Vitamin and mineral supplements: When sourcing for nutrients in your body after getting a Vertical Sleeve Gastrectomy, your best bet is the food you eat. However, because of the limited amount of food your body can take now, it is advised that you look to vitamin and minerals supplements during this period.

Your healthcare professional will give you specific recommendations based on your body type, weight, and height. Apart from the recommendations you will be given by your healthcare professional, I have compiled a list of general tips:

1. Make sure your supplements are taken as close to your mealtime as possible because some vitamins are better absorbed when taken with food. This is one of those rare times where you can shamelessly break that no-water-with-food rule. Take a few sips to get the pill down your throat if it's a tablet or capsule.
2. Stay away from gummy vitamin supplements after the surgery. A lot of them have very high sugar content and surprisingly contain a ton of calories. Moreover, they don't even meet the 100%-200% recommended daily dosage for all vitamins and mineral supplements. However, if you like the gummy versions and happen to find one that is suitable for your nutritional needs, speak to your healthcare professional about it first so you will know if it is okay to take it or not.
3. When shopping for supplements, look for ones that are sporting the USP-verified symbol. A lot of herbal medicines and supplements are not regulated or approved by the FDA for numerous valid reasons so this symbol is there to let you know what has been tested and trusted. When you see that symbol, keep in mind that it is a high-quality product.

You can also choose to buy specialty vitamins from companies like Celebrate Vitamins or Bariatric Advantage, which produce vitamins specially for patients who have undergone weight loss surgery. Despite the convenience, these specialties are not cheap and easy to come by. So if you decide to go with the regular over-the-counter supplements, that is completely okay; but if you can, opt for specialty supplements because they are USP-verified and you won't have to deal with wondering if you are taking the correct formula or dosage.

Now that I've talked about that, let's take a look at a list of vitamins and mineral supplements that might make the list your healthcare professional will give you. Remember, always consult with them first.

Multivitamins that contain minerals, preferably in liquid or chewable form: This might be recommended for the first six months post-op. You must ensure the vitamins and minerals provide 200% of the daily recommended dosage. This is usually taken twice a day as a split dose, one at the beginning of the day and one at the end.

Vitamin D: This is usually recommended for almost everyone because almost all the patients who get cleared for the surgery seem to have a vitamin D deficiency. The dosage usually recommended by healthcare professionals is 3,000 IU daily but sometimes, more is recommended for certain patients based on baseline levels.

Calcium: This one is very important and makes the list more often than not because nobody can stress the importance of bone health enough. The recommended dosage is about 1,200mg to 1,500mg daily. It should be taken two or three times in split doses.

Iron: This particular supplement will only make the list if your iron levels seem to be low, that is, if you have anemia. Iron is a very vital ingredient in the formation of red blood cells which help us transport oxygen all over the body. Recommending iron after VSG isn't standard procedure, but it might need to be done if it looks like you really need it.

Vitamin B12: The absorption of this nutrient by the body may not be top notch anymore post-op. Think of it as one of the side effects of getting sleeved. Vitamin b12 is vital for the prevention of anemia. It also ensures your nerve function is a hundred percent. Make sure to always check your routine post-op test results to know if you ever need some extra b12. The normal dosage is 1000 mcg tablets daily or through injection.

The point here is the nature of the Vertical Sleeve Gastrectomy requires a little extra help when it comes to vitamin and mineral supplementation. This commitment is for life, unfortunately, but some people don't seem to accept this fact. I have witnessed some major vitamin deficiencies in people who finally reached their weight goal and decided they didn't need the supplements anymore. They do. You do, too, and for life. You need to help your body by doing your bit. You also have to get regular blood tests to make sure you're not developing any deficiencies.

The Bariatric Kitchen

After surgery, your kitchen becomes your workshop. You need to give it a makeover, so that you only ever create healthy meals. You just need some new equipment if you don't have it already. You will also need new ingredients for the new kinds of food for your new kind of life. So get excited! Next up is a table of what foods to toss and what foods to shop for.

TRASH	STACK
Vegetable oil	Extra-virgin olive oil
All-purpose flour	Whole wheat pastry flour
Sour cream	Low fat plain Greek yogurt, hummus
Processed cheese, cheese spread	Cottage cheese, natural cheese like feta, mozzarella and cheddar
Canned pre-made soups	Canned or refried beans for the preparation of homemade soups. Low-sodium broth
Hot dogs, bacon	100% natural nitrate free turkey and nitrate free chicken
Instant oatmeal packs	Unsweetened steel-cut oats, 100% old fashioned rolled oats
Fruit snacks	Fresh fruits, 100% natural applesauce, preferably unsweetened, frozen fruit, fruit cups in water or 100% natural fruit juice
Pastrami, salami and bologna	Lean roast beef, chicken, nitrate free deli-sliced turkey, ham
Juice	Herbal tea, fresh lemons, lemon slices in water

Potato chips and pretzels	Kale chips, dehydrated snap or vegetable peas like lentil snaps or snapea crisps
Flavored regular yogurt	Low-sugar Greek yogurt, plain yogurt
Canned sausages or meats with high fat content	Canned chicken breast, shrimp, salmon, tuna packets, crabs
Pasta	Spiralized zucchini, fresh spaghetti squash
Creamy processed salad dressings	Yogurt based dressing, flavored vinegar, extra-virgin olive oil

Foods to Avoid After Surgery

The whole point of undergoing VSG is to finally experience a normal life which includes eating the right foods in moderate amounts long-term. One of the major fears patients express pre-op is the fear of intense abdominal cramps or vomiting often after the procedure.

This is a valid fear as these complications do happen, but for the first three months post-op, you should steer clear of certain foods to ensure none of these things happen to you. After three months, you can begin to slowly incorporate them back into your diet as you adjust to your new stomach. Here's what to avoid completely in the beginning:

Liquids: All sugary beverages, alcohol, fruit juices, carbonated beverages (sodas), and caffeinated beverages.

Proteins: Any breaded proteins, deep fried proteins, dry and tough meat, tough poultry.

Carbohydrates: This should be avoided completely for the first few weeks, but over the course of three months, avoid these in particular: Dried fruits, rice, fresh pineapple, all dry fiber-packed cereals like bran and granola cereal, doughy bread, pasta, popcorn, skin-on fruits.

Fats: Raw seeds or nuts, all skin-on poultry, meat with visible fat, sticky nut butters like peanut butter, fried foods, oily foods.

Food Texture Week by Week

The rate at which your diet progresses post-op should be determined by your healthcare professional. That being said, I do have a list of general guidelines for what you can expect. Keep in mind that a lot of people transition back to food with normal consistency in about 6 to 8 weeks after the surgery.

Post-op Diet Timeline

- First and second day - Clear liquid diet
- First to second week - Full liquid diet
- Third week - Pureed food
- Fourth to six week - Soft foods
- Seventh to eight week - Transition back to normal food

Chapter 4: Early Post-Op Foods

High-Protein Milk

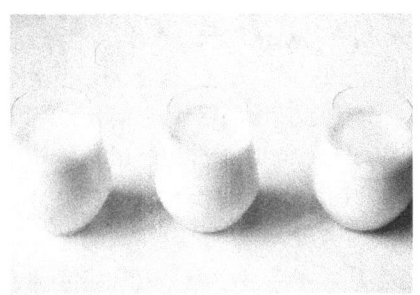

- Prep time: 5 minutes
- Cooking time: 0 minutes
- Serving: 4
- Calories: 144kcal per serving
- Fat: 0g|Carbs: 21g|Protein: 14g

This costs roughly 40 cents per cup to get together and it hits you with an entire 14g of protein. This is just a way of saying that you do not need all the fancy protein powders to get as much protein as your body needs during this period. This recipe can be used to make a nice cup of milk that can be drank by itself or used in the preparation of a protein drink. It can also be used as a substitute for milk when cooking. This drink should definitely make your meal plan list after VSG!

INGREDIENTS

1. Nonfat dry milk powder (1 cup)
2. Skim milk (4 cups)

INSTRUCTIONS

1. Pour milk and milk powder into a deep bowl and whisk very slowly until the milk powder is completely dissolved and invisible. If you happen not to own a manual whisk, you can use a blender. Just pour the skim milk and powder into the blender and pulse on high for 6 minutes or until everything is thoroughly mixed.
2. That's all that is needed. Serve immediately then store the excess in an airtight cup or bowl and place in the refrigerator. Just like most leftovers, the flavor blends and becomes enhanced overnight. This recipe can only keep for about 7 days. Discard any remainder after that time.

Note: Milk is an amazing source of protein, minerals and vitamins. It is very important for the healing process post-op and the weight loss that follows. You might be wondering if you can just substitute this for plant based milk instead. That decision is up to you and your healthcare professional, but I will tell you what I do know.

Plant-based milks are usually packed with various important nutrients, but one thing they all lack is the amount of protein contained in cow's milk. Examples of plant based milks are coconut milk, rice milk, soy milk, almond milk, hemp milk, etc.

Soy milk is a bit different from the rest because it contains almost as much protein as the typical cow's milk. Soy milk can contain about 6g to 7g of protein per cup. Keep in mind that all milk products contain some amount of natural sugar.

Lactose is found in milk. This isn't found in other food and beverages packed with added sugar. You see, lactose belongs to a class of carbohydrates called "disaccharides" and your body will have to break it down first before digesting and absorbing it. Some people have a condition called lactose intolerance which means the inability of the body to break down lactose. Most of them avoid milk and milk products completely, others opt for lactose-free milk or get lactase medications that provide them with the enzyme needed to break down lactose.

Pumpkin Spice Latte Protein Shake

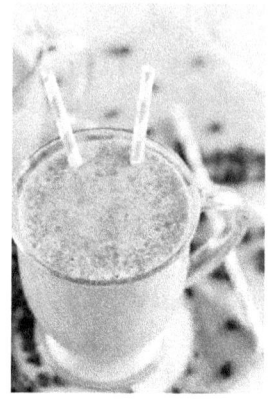

- Prep time: 5 minutes
- Cooking time: 0 minutes
- Serving: 2
- Calories: 125kcal per serving
- Fat: 0g|Carbs: 12g|Protein: 15g

This recipe reminds me of the fall season poured into a glass in the form of a beverage. You have the sweet pumpkin, dear old nutmeg, heartwarming coffee and everyone's favorite, cinnamon! This drink is promised to satisfy your autumn longing for a pumpkin spiced lattes but from the comfort of your kitchen. Oh, you also get to toss all that artificial sugar and bad fat!

INGREDIENTS

1. Cinnamon powder (1 teaspoon)
2. Nutmeg powder or ground nutmeg seed (¼ teaspoon)
3. Nonfat milk or soy milk, unsweetened (1 cup)
4. Ground ginger or ginger powder (¼ teaspoon)
5. Decaffeinated coffee, brewed (¾ cup)
6. Ground cloves (⅛ teaspoon)
7. Vanilla flavored protein powder (¼ cup)

INSTRUCTIONS

1. Pour the pumpkin puree, coffee, milk, protein powder, cloves, ginger, nutmeg and cinnamon into a blender. Pulse on high heat for about 3 minutes or until you see that the powder has completely dissolved to produce a smooth mixture.
2. Get a glass and fill it halfway. Enjoy your tasty pumpkin shake.
3. Store any leftovers in an airtight bowl immediately and refrigerate for later. It can keep for about a week. Don't forget to blend it first before serving

Notes: You can make a customized pumpkin pie spice and use it to make smoothies, baked squash or even oatmeal. It can also be used to add flavor to plain Greek yogurt. For the customized spice, all you need is:

1. Cinnamon powder (2 tablespoons)
2. Ground cloves (½ teaspoon)
3. Ginger powder (1 teaspoon)
4. Ground allspice (½ teaspoon)
5. Nutmeg powder (1 teaspoon)

Mix them together and store for later in an airtight container.

Double Fudge Chocolate Shake

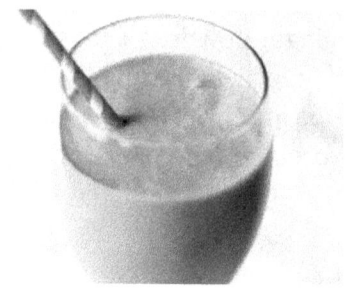

- Prep time: 5 minutes
- Cooking time: 5 minutes
- Serving: 2
- Calories: 157kcal per serving
- Fats: 1g|Carbs: 18g|Protein: 20g

Who doesn't love chocolate or chocolate-flavored anything? Personally, I love chocolate so much that it has its own food group on my menu. There are fruits, protein, dairy, veggies and grains, then there is chocolate. Getting sleeved might mean forfeiting a lot of tasty desserts, but not this one.

Chocolate is fine only when eaten right. By right, I mean the healthy kinds and in the right amounts. This recipe is made with cocoa powder, but the unsweetened version which means you get the chocolate minus the added sugar.

INGREDIENTS

1. Low fat plain Greek yogurt (½ cup)
2. Banana (½ small size)
3. Low fat milk or soy milk, unsweetened (1 cup)
4. Chocolate protein powder (¼ cup)
5. Vanilla extract (½ teaspoon)
6. Cocoa powder, unsweetened (2 tablespoons)

INSTRUCTIONS

1. Pour the yogurt, cocoa powder, milk, vanilla extract, protein powder, yogurt and banana into a blender and pulse on high for about 3 minutes or until you notice that the powders have completely dissolved to produce a smooth paste.
2. As usual, get a glass and serve yourself half a cup of the shake. I hope you enjoy it.
3. All leftovers must be stored in an airtight container in the refrigerator for about a week. That's how long it will last.

Notes: We all know chocolate is gotten from cacao or cocoa beans. There are two kinds of baking cocoa; the unsweetened cocoa powder and the Dutch-process cocoa powder. When shopping for groceries, keep an out for the 100% unsweetened cocoa powder. It tastes a little more acidic than the Dutch-process kind but it is definitely healthier, containing flavonols and antioxidants. Paying close attention to the kind of cocoa required for a particular recipe is very important because something as simple as that can change the entire taste of whatever you make.

Protein-Packed Peanut Butter Cup Shake

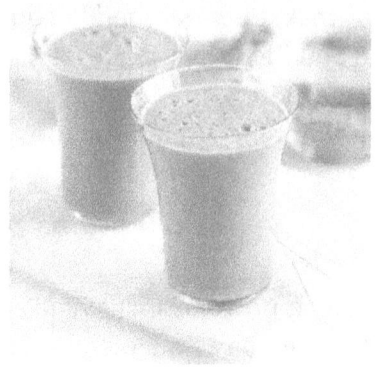

- Prep time: 5 minutes
- Cooking time: 0 minutes
- Serving: 2
- Calories: 215kcal per serving
- Fats: 3g | Carbs: 18g | Protein: 27g

It shouldn't exactly come as a surprise to you that Reese's peanut butter cups are among the best-selling candies all over the world. Why this is, is because of the sweet chocolate exterior and creamy peanut butter in the middle. That taste is pretty hard to be unaffected by and I know that this candy is strictly off limits to sleeved patients, but it doesn't mean you have to live and die with unsatisfied cravings, not while I'm here. This protein shake is everything you have been searching for and more. It is absolutely tasty and protein packed so you don't get to lose anything when you give into your sweet tooth. If you have time this afternoon, give this a go. You'll find that you don't think about the candy jar very often anymore.

INGREDIENTS:

1. Low fat plain Greek yogurt (½ cup)
2. Chocolate protein powder (¼ cup)
3. Low fat milk (1 cup)
4. Cocoa powder (2 tablespoons)
5. Nonfat ricotta cheese (¼ cup)
6. Peanut butter powder (2 tablespoons)

INSTRUCTIONS

1. Pour the ricotta cheese, peanut butter powder, milk, cocoa powder, yogurt, and protein powder into a blender and pulse on high for about 4 minutes or until all the powders are well dissolved to produce a smooth mixture.
2. Serve yourself a half filled glass of this protein shake.
3. Place any leftovers in an airtight bowl immediately and store it in the fridge. It can keep for a week. Don't forget to blend before serving.

Notes: Peanut butter is no doubt one of the good guys in the fat family, but one thing you should keep in mind is how calorie-packed it also is. Be careful with portions because a simple tablespoon of peanut butter carries a whole 90 calories. When shopping for groceries, stay on the lookout for natural peanut butter versions. They don't contain added palm oil, which is a saturated fat or artificial sugars. Another thing you can do is pour peanut butter powder into a bowl and add water. Mix it thoroughly to make your own spread for oatmeal. Peanut butter powder has a very high protein content but has less calorie content.

Vanilla Apple Pie Protein Shake

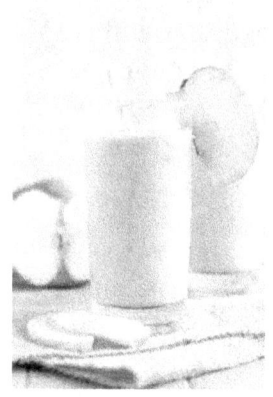

- Prep time: 5 minutes
- Cooking time: 0 minutes
- Serving: 2
- Calories: 123kcal per serving
- Fat: 1g|Carbs: 14g|Protein: 14g

Tell me something more satisfying than fresh apple pie and ice cream. I'll wait. This particular dessert is a classic and with it comes feelings of warmth and joy. This recipe hits me with a lot of good memories from granny's house. This apple pie shake is the VSG version of the regular dessert that I'm sure you miss but not for long. It tastes just like apple pie, but it contains less calories than apple pie so you get to keep that trim waistline after all.

INGREDIENTS

1. Vanilla protein powder (¼ cup)
2. Cinnamon powder (2 teaspoons)
3. Ice cubes
4. Low fat milk (1 cup)
5. Diced, cored apple, skinless (1 small)
6. Nutmeg powder (½ teaspoon)
7. Vanilla extract (1 teaspoon)

INSTRUCTIONS

1. Pour the apple, cinnamon powder, milk, vanilla extract, nutmeg powder, protein powder and ice cubes into a blender and pulse on high for 5 minutes or until you see that all the powders have been dissolved and you have a smooth mixture.
2. Serve yourself a half filled glass of the protein shake and enjoy.
3. Any leftovers must be poured into an airtight bowl and placed in the fridge immediately. They will keep for a week, after that, it should be disposed of. Don't forget to blend before serving.

Tropical Mango Smoothie

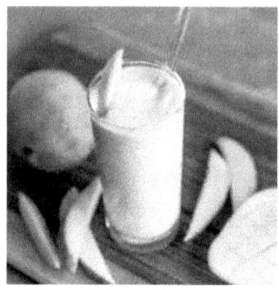

- Prep time: 5 minutes
- Cooking time: 0 minutes
- Serving: 2
- Calories: 115kcal per serving
- Fats: 2.5g | Carbs: 9g | Protein: 15g

Fruit smoothies are everything we need on a typical hot day in the summer. I prefer to have this one at the beach or when lounging in my backyard or by the pool. Smoothies are so tasty that it is tempting to just chug over a thousand calories in the form of these sugary beverages.

Most smoothies contain so many calories because a lot of them are not as 100% natural as they claim to be. This recipe however, happens to be the real deal. At least, you get to see the fruits yourself before getting out as much juice as you can and sipping away. Ever wanted to go to the beach but not to the beach? Sip this, lay back and close your eyes.

INGREDIENTS

1. Frozen mango chunks (¼ cup)
2. Low fat plain Greek yogurt (½ cup)
3. Vanilla protein powder (¼ cup)
4. Canned pineapple chunks soaked in 100% all natural juice or water (¼ cup)
5. Coconut milk, unsweetened or low fat milk (1 cup)
6. Ice cubes

INSTRUCTIONS

1. Pour the protein powder, pineapple chunks, milk, yogurt, mango and ice cubed into a blender and pulse on high for about 4 minutes or until you see a smooth paste with no visible powders.
2. Serve yourself a half filled glass of this goodness.
3. All leftovers should be poured into an airtight container and placed in the refrigerator. They will keep for a week. Don't forget to blend before serving.

Notes: When shopping for fruits, go straight to the freezer section for the good stuff. Frozen fruits bring their own charm to the table. They add a certain thickness to the protein shake or smoothie without needing to use extra ice. If you're looking for fruits that are not currently in season, the frozen section might have what you're looking for. Plus you don't have to be worried about your fruits going bad over time because they keep very well in the freezer for quite a while. You know the drill: 100% natural fruits always.

Chapter 5: Breakfast Recipes

Smoothie Bowl With Greek Yogurt And Fresh Berries

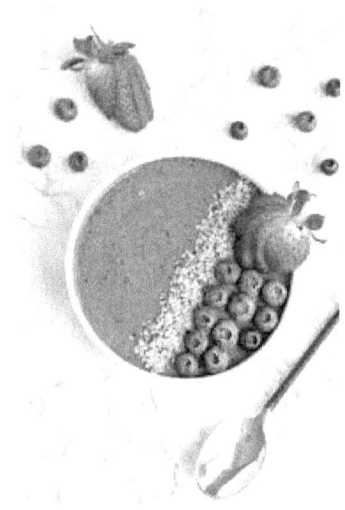

- Prep time: 5 minutes
- Cooking time: 10 minutes
- Serving: 1
- Calories: 255kcal per serving
- Fats: 10g|Carbs: 21g|Protein: 20g

Meals are more than just the taste. It has a lot to do with how the meals look and where we eat said meals. All these factors have a major impact on feelings 9f satiety after a meal. What some people don't realize is that having your meals in a stress-packed environment and having the same meal in a more serene familiar environment will affect a person differently.

These factors can determine whether or not a food makes you sick. Next time you want to have breakfast fast, don't quickly gulp down a glass of protein shake while rushing out of the house. Instead, consider settling down to enjoy this homemade nutrient packed smoothie bowl. Your eyes will love it as much as your taste buds will, I promise!

INGREDIENTS

1. Vanilla flavored almond milk, unsweetened or low fat milk (¾ cup)
2. Vanilla or plain protein powder (⅛ cup)
3. Fresh raspberries (¼ cup)
4. Fresh spinach (⅓ cup)
5. Frozen mixed berries (¼ cup)
6. Low fat plain Greek yogurt (¼ cup)
7. Fresh blueberries (¼ cup)
8. Chia seeds (1 teaspoon)
9. Almond slivers (1 tablespoon)

INSTRUCTIONS

1. Pour the milk, protein powder, yogurt, frozen berries and spinach into a blender and pulse on high for about 4 minutes or until everything looks thoroughly blended.
2. Transfer the mixture into a serving bowl and garnish with blueberries, chia seeds, raspberries and almonds. That's it! Eat with a spoon.

Notes: This is just one variation of this recipe. It can be garnished with a lot of different fruits for a different flavor. Change up the toppings every once in a while so you don't get bored. There's a mango-pineapple version, you should try it. Garnish with unsweetened coconut flakes.

Cherry-Vanilla Baked Oatmeal

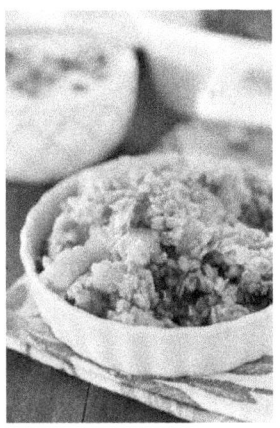

- Prep time: 10 minutes
- Cooking time: 45 minutes
- Serving: 6
- Calories: 149kcal per serving
- Fats: 4g | Carbs: 21g | Protein: 8g

When we go to the coffee shop, we like to grab a pastry on the way out, something sweet and not necessarily filling. That's a no-go zone for you now that you have gotten sleeved but don't be sad. Why bother about coffee shop pastries when you can make your own even healthier versions? Look no farther, darlings. This baked oatmeal recipe is the answer to all your questions. No need for the fat-filled, calorie-packed ones of the past. This can be prepared for breakfast on Sunday and the leftovers can be preserved and had the rest of the week.

INGREDIENTS

1. Eggs (3 medium)
2. Old-fashioned oats (1 cup)
3. Flaxseed powder (1 tablespoon)
4. Vanilla extract (1 teaspoon)
5. Cinnamon powder (½ teaspoon)
6. Low-fat milk (1 cup)
7. Liquid stevia (1 teaspoon)
8. Baking powder (¾ teaspoon)
9. Diced cored skinless apples (1 medium)

Low fat plain Greek yogurt (½ cup)

Fresh cherries with the pits removed (1 cup)

Nonstick cooking spray

INSTRUCTIONS

1. Prepare your oven. Preheat to 375°F. Grease an 8-by-8 inch baking dish with nonstick cooking spray.
2. Get a medium bowl. Pour in cinnamon powder, flaxseed, oats and baking powder into it. Mix thoroughly and set aside.
3. In a much larger bowl, crack the eggs and whisk. Then add yogurt, stevia, milk and vanilla. Whisk again until thoroughly mixed.
4. Stir the dry ingredients into the wet ingredients. Now pour in diced apples and cherries then gently fold them into the mixture.
5. Pour mixture into prepared baking dish and slide it into the oven to bake. Leave it for about 45 minutes or until you notice the edges pulling away from the walls of the pan and the oatmeal bouncing back when poked.

6. Place any leftovers into airtight glass bowls and place them in the fridge. They will keep for a week. Microwave before serving

Notes: Play around with the extras in the oatmeal. In fact, make the recipes seasonal even. Change it up every now and then. Use pumpkin puree in place of the yogurt. Use unsweetened dried cranberries instead of the usual cherries if you'd like a nice holiday twist. Place the apples and cherries on the shelf and replace them with 100% natural fresh berries. If you'd like a super creamy consistency, I would like to suggest adding a quarter cup of low-fat milk when serving

High-Protein Pancakes

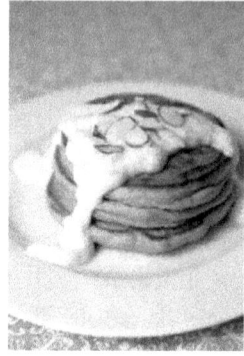

- Prep time: 5 minutes
- Cooking time: 5 minutes
- Serving: 4
- Calories: 182kcal per serving
- Fats: 10g|Carbs: 1og|Protein: 12g

Hungry for some Saturday morning flapjacks that don't come with all the artificial sugar and processed carbs? Say no more! These high protein pancakes are all you need to start the weekend. The ingredients for these recipes are very obtainable. You might even have some or all in your refrigerator or pantry.

INGREDIENTS

1. Melted coconut oil (1 ½ tablespoons)
2. Eggs (3 medium)
3. Whole wheat pastry flour (⅓ cup)
4. Nonstick cooking spray

5. Low fat cottage cheese (1 cup)

INSTRUCTIONS

1. Gently beat the eggs in a large bowl.
2. Stir in flour, coconut oil and cottage cheese until thoroughly mixed.
3. Place a large pan over medium-low heat and grease the pan with a single coat of cooking spray.
4. You will need a measuring cup for this part. Drizzle about ⅓ cup of pancake batter into greased pan and leave it to cook for about 3 minutes or until you notice air bubbles on top of the pancake.
5. Flip the pancakes to cook the other side until it looks golden brown. This should take about 2 minutes. Take it out of the pan and repeat the process until the batter is finished.
6. Serve warm

Notes: For toppings, you can use plain Greek yogurt, sugar-free syrup, fresh berries or unsweetened applesauce. You can experiment with 100% natural peanut butter and bananas when you have transitioned back to a regular diet.

Southwestern Scrambled Eggs Burritos

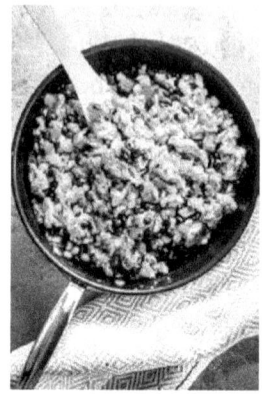

- Prep time: 10 minutes
- Cooking time: 10 minutes
- Serving: 8
- Calories: 250kcal per serving
- Fats: 10g|Carbs: 28g|Protein: 19g

Burritos, a crowd pleaser! If you're scared of having burritos because of all the fat and artificial sodium, fear no more. This recipe will leave you completely satisfied and still in the clear. They can be prepared and stored ahead of time. Makes for a quick hot and healthy breakfast.

INGREDIENTS

1. Extra-virgin olive oil (1 teaspoon)
2. Chopped red bell pepper (1 medium)

3. Chopped green bell pepper (1 medium)
4. Low fat milk (¼ cup)
5. Whole wheat tortillas (8 medium)
6. Eggs (12 small)
7. Drained and rinsed black beans (1 can)
8. Salsa (1 cup
9. Diced onion (½ medium)

INSTRUCTIONS

1. Mix the eggs and milk in a large bowl.
2. Place a large pan over medium heat and drizzle olive oil onto it. Pour in bell peppers and onions then stir fry for about 3 minutes or until it softens. Stir in the beans.
3. Pour in the milk mixture and lower the heat to a simmer and gently stir with a silicone spatula for roughly 4 minutes or until the eggs look cooked through and fluffy.
4. Place the tortillas on a clean flat surface and scoop the scrambled egg mixture onto each of them. Fold the tortilla. Bottom end first, then the sides then roll.
5. Serve warm with a side of salsa. Place any leftovers in the fridge to preserve. This will keep for a week. To serve, microwave for 1 minute and 30 seconds. If you want to store them for longer than a week, you will have to put them on ice.

Notes: If you would like more veggies in your meal, get a bag of frozen all natural mixed vegetables at the grocery store. Place a greased skillet over medium heat and stir fry the vegetables before adding the eggs. That's it!

Hearty Slow Cooker Cinnamon Oatmeal

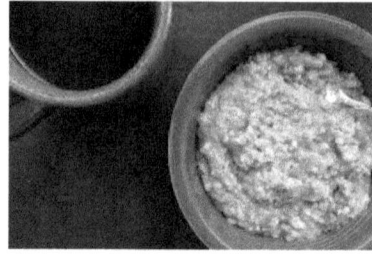

- Prep time: 5 minutes
- Cooking time: 8 hours
- Serving: 10
- Calories: 136kcal
- Fats: 2g | Carbs: 23g | Protein: 6g

The National Weight Control Registry has said that having regular breakfast is crucial to weight loss and should be made a habit. However, the reality is that it is really hard to not miss breakfast sometimes for so many valid reasons, but this recipe is here to fix all that. With this recipe, you can cook your breakfast a day before and preserve leftovers for the rest of the week.

INGREDIENTS

1. Steel-cut oats (2 cups)
2. Nutmeg powder (1 teaspoon)
3. Water (8 cups)
4. Cinnamon powder (2 teaspoons)

Protein add-ins (Use one at a time)

1. Vanilla or unflavored protein powder (2 tablespoons)
2. Peanut butter powder (2 tablespoons)
3. Low fat milk (½ cup)
4. Nonfat milk powder or powdered egg white (2 tablespoons)

Protein add-ins for 8 weeks post-op

1. Pumpkin puree (¼ cup)
2. Frozen or fresh berries (½ cup)
3. Chopped walnuts, almonds or pecans (⅛ cup)
4. Peeled pear, banana, apple or pear slices (½ medium)

INSTRUCTIONS

1. Pour oats, water, nutmeg and cinnamon powder into a slow cooker. Put a lid on it and place it over l9w heat to simmer for about 8 hours or 7, give or take.
2. You have quite a number of protein add-ins to pick from. Choose one and stir it into the mixture right before serving. Feel free to change it up anytime you like.

Notes: A quick tip, oatmeal is packed with soluble fiber needed for topnotch heart health. All foods that contain soluble fiber have been tested and trusted to reduce the bad cholesterol in your blood leading to a healthy heart and healthier you. If you're in need of a quick, healthy and filling breakfast, go for oatmeal.

Mini Bariatric Sized Meatloaf

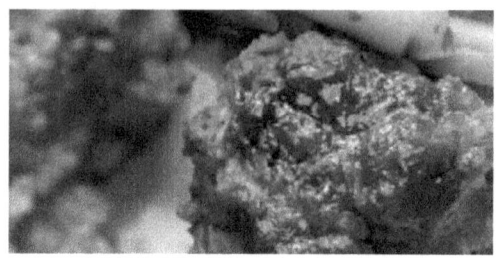

- Prep time: 10 minutes
- Cooking time: 35 minutes
- Serving: 12 mini
- Calories: 110kcal
- Fats: 5g|Carbs: 9g|Protein: 11g

INGREDIENTS

1. Salt (1 ¼ teaspoons)
2. Finely chopped green bell pepper (½ cup)
3. 93% lean ground beef (1lb)
4. Egg substitute (½ cup)
5. Black pepper powder (¼ teaspoon)
6. Shredded parmesan cheese (½ cup)
7. Finely diced onion (½ cup)
8. Low sugar ketchup (2 tablespoons)
9. Chopped tomatoes (8 oz)

INSTRUCTIONS

1. First things first, prepare your oven. Set it to 375°F. Spray an even layer of cooking spray onto some muffin tins.
2. Pour onion, ground beef, bell pepper, egg, salt, pepper, and parmesan cheese into a bowl. Pour the diced tomatoes and just enough of the juice to get the perfect consistency. Don't make it too moist or it might fall apart.
3. Wash your hands thoroughly and use it to mix the contents of the bowl thoroughly.
4. Pour mixture into greased muffin pan and drizzle ketchup on top.
5. Slide it into the oven to bake for about 35 minutes.
6. Serve warm.

Chapter 6: Lunch Recipes

Bashed Chicken With Tomatoes, Olives, And Capers

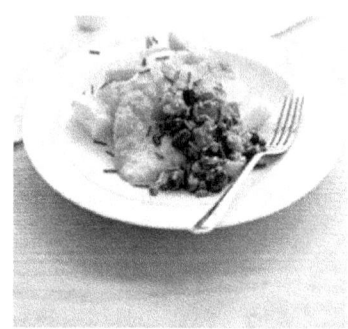

- Prep time: 5 minutes
- Cooking time: 40 minutes
- Serving: 2
- Calories: 247kcal
- Fats: 10g|Carbs: 5g|Protein: 28g

INGREDIENTS

1. Low fat nonstick cooking spray
2. Capers (2 teaspoons)
3. Boneless chicken breast, skinned (1 small)
4. Finely diced ripe tomatoes (1 large)
5. Seasoned flour, almond flour or ground almonds, shredded parmesan cheese (1 tablespoon)
6. Ripe or black olives (6 small)
7. Finely chopped parsley or fresh chives (1 teaspoon)

8. White wine, water, bouillon/chicken stock (For this recipe, stock was used)

INSTRUCTIONS

1. Slice the chicken breast horizontally into half. Well, not completely. Just slice it enough so it can be spread open like a book. Use a meat tenderizer to bash the meat. If you don't own a tenderizer, try using a rolling pin.
2. Pour almond flour or ground almonds, parmesan cheese or seasoned flour into a bowl and toss the chicken breast into the bowl to coat.
3. Grease a skillet with low fat cooking spray. Be generous with it. Place it over medium heat and place the coated chicken in it for 4 minutes per side or until it looks golden brown and cooked through. Take it out of the pan and set it aside.
4. Now pour the tomatoes, olives and capers into the pan and stir in liquid of preference (white wine, water or bouillon). Now sprinkle seasoning into the pan and mix thoroughly. Leave it to boil, then reduce the heat to simmer for 4 minutes or until you notice the tomatoes starting to break down.
5. Serve the chicken on a plate and pour tomato mixture over it. Garnish with parsley.

Gingered Ham

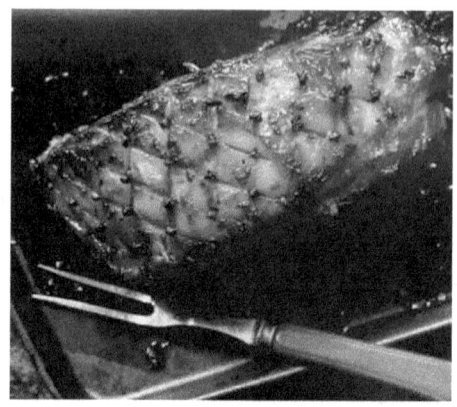

- Prep time: 20 minutes
- Cooking time: 5 hours
- Serving: 8
- Calories: 470kcal
- Fat: 23.4g|Carbs: 2.6g|Protein: 64g

Say hello to this flavor-filled slow cooked ham. This oven-cooked goodness is super soft meat with a sticky glaze that melts in your mouth. Definitely a crowd favorite, this can be prepared for special occasions or just lunch.

INGREDIENTS

1. Quartered onion (1 medium)
2. Boneless gammon joint, unsmoked (3kg)

3. Black peppercorns (10 medium)
4. Sugar-free ginger beer (2 ½ cups)
5. Sliced skinless ginger root (1 small)
6. Shredded ginger root (1 tablespoon)
7. Low sugar jelly, orange conserve marmalade or ginger jam (3 tablespoons)
8. Whole cloves (6 medium)
9. Extra cloves for garnish

INSTRUCTION

1. Prepare the oven. Heat to 325°F or gas 3.
2. To cook the ham, place it in a deep roasting pan that is big enough to hold the joint.
3. Now pour in all of the ginger beer except ⅓ cup of it. Add the onion, peppercorns, cloves and ginger to the ham mixture.
4. Use two layers of foil to cover the pan and place it in the oven for about 4½ hours.
5. Now remove the foil and drain all the juices except 1 tablespoon.
6. Raise the oven temperature to 400°F or gas 6.
7. To prepare the glaze, pour the leftover ginger beer, ginger jam and shredded ginger into a saucepan and let it boil.
8. Lower the heat and leave it to simmer for about 5 minutes or until it starts to look like a syrup.
9. Don't forget to peel off all the skin from the ham, sparing just a little bit of fat.

Use a small knife to make a diamond pattern onto the fat and then apply as much glaze as you want over the decor.

Feel free to add studded cloves to the decoration before putting it back into the oven to cook without a lid for just 10 minutes.

Apply some more glaze and let it cook for an extra 15 minutes or until it looks brown.

10. Serve warm.

Lamb And Crispy Potato Hot Pot

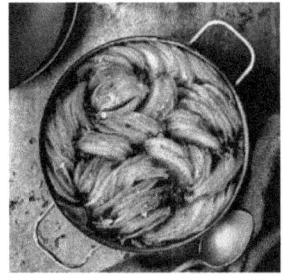

- Prep time: 15 minutes
- Cooking time: 2 hours, 45 minutes
- Serving: 6
- Calories: 300kcal
- Fats: 6.2g|Carbs: 29g|Protein: 32g

INGREDIENTS

1. Thinly sliced onions (2 small)
2. Black pepper powder
3. Salt
4. Low fat nonstick cooking spray
5. Diced carrots (2 medium)
6. Plain flour (1 tablespoon)
7. Extra lean chopped lamb (700g)
8. Worcestershire sauce (2 teaspoons)
9. Baby potatoes (750g)

Lamb stock or meat stock (2 ¼ cups)

Bay leaves (2 medium)

Fresh thyme leaves (2 sprigs)

INSTRUCTIONS

1. Generously grease a casserole dish with some low fat cooking spray. The casserole dish must have a lid.
2. Generously spritz a large lidded casserole with low-fat cooking spray or mist. Add the onions, carrots and lamb and fry for 5-8 minutes until the meat is browned. Season to taste with salt and pepper.
3. Add the flour and stir well to coat and cook for 1 minute. Gradually add the stock with the Worcestershire sauce and bay leaves and bring to the boil. Reduce the heat, cover and cook for 20 minutes.
4. Preheat the oven to 200 C/400 F/gas 6.
5. Meanwhile, very thinly slice the potatoes ideally using a mandolin or very finely and arrange into short stacks.
6. Take the lid off the casserole and arrange the potato slices upright on top, fitting closely together to create swirling patterns. Spritz generously with low-fat cooking spray or mist, season with salt and pepper and sprinkle with half of the fresh thyme.
7. Cover the dish and cook in the oven for 1½ hours. Remove the lid and cook for a further 45 minutes, or until potatoes are browned.
8. Serve sprinkled with the remaining thyme to serve.

Rosti-Style Herder's Pie

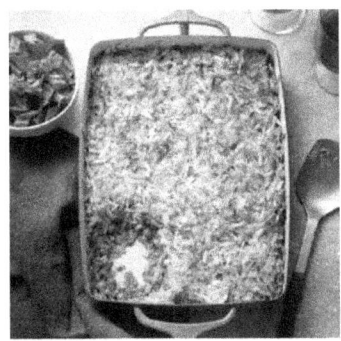

- Prep time: 20 minutes
- Cooking time: 1 hour 40 minutes
- Serving: 6
- Calories: 270kcal
- Fats: 20g | Carbs: 20.4g | Protein: 31.1g

INGREDIENTS

1. Finely diced onion (1 large)
2. Beef stock/bouillon (1 cube)
3. Extra lean minced or ground beef (800g)
4. Passata or creamed tomatoes (1 ¼ cups)
5. Frozen peas (1 handful)
6. Worcestershire sauce (3 tablespoons)
7. Shredded carrots (1 medium)
8. Black pepper powder
9. Salt

Shredded skinless sweet potato (1 medium)

Shredded parsnips (2 medium)

Low-fat nonstick cooking spray

INSTRUCTION

1. Prepare your oven. Preheat to 300°F.
2. Now you're going to place the beef in a nonstick pan and leave to cook until both sides look golden brown. Sprinkle the onions into the pan and cook for an extra 10 minutes until it's tender.
3. Stir in the passata. Sprinkle the stock cube, pepper and salt then pour in the Worcestershire sauce. Mix thoroughly and leave to cook for roughly 5 minutes.
4. Now cover the pan and place it in the oven to cook for about 1 hour.
5. Now raise the heat to 400°F and add frozen peas.
6. Pour the sweet potatoes, carrots and parsnips into a bowl then coat with cooking spray and mix.
7. Use the veggie mix to coat the meat mixture. Place a foil over the pan and put it back into the oven to bake for about 20 minutes.
8. Now take off the foil and let the pie cook for about 15 minutes or until the top is golden brown and crisp.
9. Let the pie sit for 10 minutes before you serve.

Notes: Cabbages or cooked spring beans go well with this pie

California Burger

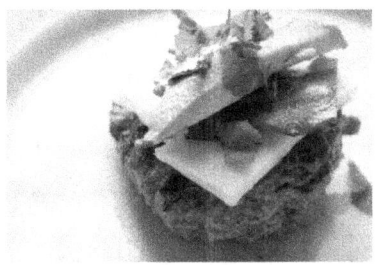

- Prep time: 10 minutes
- Cooking time: 20 minutes
- Serving: 6
- Calories:
- Fat: 9g | Carbs: 2g | Protein: 21g

INGREDIENTS

1. Sliced avocado (¼ medium)
2. 93% lean ground beef (1lb)
3. Low fat pepper jack cheese (3 slices)
4. Salt (¼ teaspoon)
5. Pepper (¼ teaspoon)
6. Maple turkey or regular bacon (3 strips)
7. Finely chopped cilantro (1 tablespoon)

INSTRUCTIONS

1. Make 4 patties with the ground beef. Preheat q grill. Set it to medium.

2. Season each side of all the patties and place them on the grill to cook. Leave it to cook for 5 minutes then flip to cook the other side for another 5 minutes.
3. While the patties are cooking, place the turkey bacon in a different pan for just 4 minutes, flipping only once.
4. Cut the avocado into slices and cut the cilantro.
5. All the ingredients should be ready now. Start setting up the burgers. To do this, you'll have to place the bottom half of the burger on a place and place half a slice of cheese on it. Layer with half slice of turkey bacon, a slice of avocado and chopped cilantro.

Chapter 7: Vegetarian Recipes

Roasted Vegetable Quinoa Salad With Chickpeas

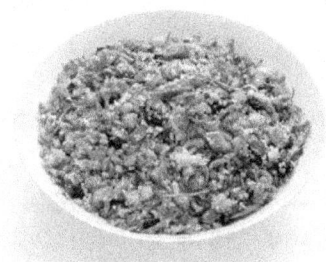

- Prep time: 15 minutes
- Cooking time: 30 minutes
- Serving: 6
- Calories: 200kcal
- Fats: 9g | Carbs: 27g | Protein: 7g

INGREDIENTS

1. Diced zucchini (1 small)
2. Low sodium chicken or vegetable stock (1 cup)
3. Diced eggplant (1 small)
4. Dried basil (1 tablespoon)
5. Diced yellow summer squash (1 small)
6. Extra virgin olive oil (3 tablespoons)
7. Minced fresh garlic (1 teaspoon)

8. Halved grape tomatoes (½ cup)
9. Fresh lemon juice (2 tablespoons)

Drained and rinsed chickpeas (1 can)

Packaged quinoa (⅓ cup)

Dried oregano (1 teaspoon)

INSTRUCTIONS

1. First things first, prepare your oven. Heat to 425°F.
2. Get a sheet pan ready by lining it with parchment paper.
3. Now place the zucchini, tomatoes, eggplant, chickpeas and yellow squash on the baking sheet. Spread them out and then drizzle 1 tablespoon of olive oil into the pan. Toss to coat.
4. Slide the pan into the oven to bake for about 30 minutes. Stir only once. When it is ready, it should be soft and juicy. Not the chickpeas though, those will be crisp and firm.
5. You can do other things while the veggies roast. Place a small saucepan over medium heat and pour in stock and quinoa. Place the lid on the pan and leave it to boil. Once it is boiling, lower the heat and leave it to simmer for just 15 minutes. You should find that all the liquid has been absorbed. Turn off the heat and use a fork to fluff the quinoa. Set aside
6. Get a small bowl. Pour un garlic, 2 tablespoons of olive oil and lemon juice. Mix thoroughly. Now stir in oregano and basil until thoroughly mixed.
7. To serve, mix the quinoa, veggies and garlic dressing. Stir very gently. Enjoy!

Notes: if you would like to increase the protein content of this recipe, just serve with lean grilled chicken breast or a piece of baked fish. Feel free to scoop some low-fat plain Greek yogurt onto the mixture.

Mexican Stuffed Summer Squash

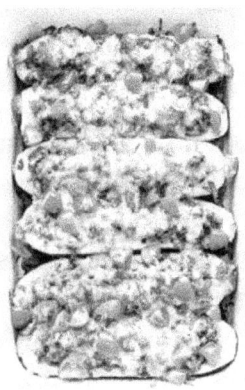

- Prep time: 5 minutes
- Cooking time: 33 minutes
- Serving: 2
- Calories: 190kcal
- Fats: 8g|Carbs: 21g|Protein: 9g

INGREDIENTS

1. Yellow summer squash (1 medium)
2. Cooked quinoa (½ cup)
3. Diced tomato (1 small)
4. Refried black beans (½ cup)
5. Grated Colby jack cheese (¼ cup)
6. Chopped scallions (2 small)

7. Nonstick cooking spray
8. Chopped black olives (2 tablespoons)

INSTRUCTIONS

1. Prepare your oven. Preheat to 400°F.
2. Grease an 8-by-8-inch baking dish with enough cooking spray.
3. Remove and dispose of the ends of the summer squash. Slice it in half horizontally and then remove and dispose of the seeds with a spoon. Now put the squash on greased baking dish with the cut side down.
4. Use something small to create holes in the squash so that it can breathe. Now pour a tablespoon of water into the dish.
5. Place the baking dish in the microwave and leave it to heat for 3 minutes or until it feels soft. Bring it out and drain any excess water.
6. Leave the squash to cool until it is cold enough to touch. Now place the squash so that the cut sides are facing up and far away from each other
7. Scoop ¼ cup of beans into each squash and then layer ¼ cup of quinoa. Pour Colby jack cheese over the top and cover the dish with foil. Slide the dish into the oven to bake for about 25 minutes.
8. When 25 minutes is up, take out the foil and bake for another 5 minutes or until you see the cheese looking all bubbly.
9. For garnishing, top with olives, scallions and tomatoes right before you serve.

Notes: Don't be stingy with the extras. Change it up every now and then. A soy-based meat tossed in taco seasoning substitute will do the trick or brown ground turkey. You can also stir fry onions and bell peppers to serve with cilantro and avocado.

Barley-Mushroom Risotto

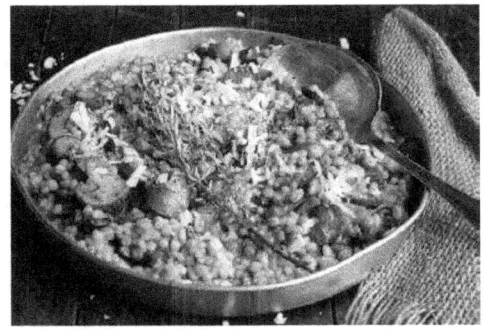

- Prep time: 5 minutes
- Cooking time: 55 minutes
- Serving: 6
- Calories: 104kcal
- Fats: 3g | Carbs: 16g | Protein: 3g

INGREDIENTS

1. Minced garlic (1 teaspoon)
2. Sliced mushrooms (4 cups)
3. Extra virgin olive oil (1 tablespoon)
4. Dry white wine (½ cup)
5. Water (1 cup)
6. Chopped whole leeks (2 medium)
7. Pearl barley (½ cup)
8. Dried thyme (2 teaspoons)
9. Low Sodium chicken or vegetable stock (1 ½ cups)
Fresh spinach leaves (3 cups)

INSTRUCTIONS

1. Heat the olive oil in a large pan set over medium heat. Pour in garlic and sauté for a minute. Stir tin the leeks and stir fry for about 3 minutes or until it's soft.
2. Pour in the mushrooms and leave it to cook until it's soft and golden brown. This should take about 4 minutes.
3. Add the barley and thyme. Stir and leave it to cook for an additional 2 minutes.
4. Pour in the wine and stir gently. Lower the heat and let it simmer for a roughly 5 minutes or until all the liquid has dried up.
5. Stir in the water and stock. Leave the heat on low, put the lid on and leave it to simmer for about 40 minutes. Don't forget to stir every once in a while to ensure the barley doesn't get stuck to the bottom of the pan.
6. Now slowly add the spinach and stir until it wilts.
7. Serve warm.

Notes: This meal isn't exactly the richest in protein despite substituting barley for rice. Mind you, barley is much richer in protein than rice. To ramp up the protein content, throw in some Parmigiano-Reggiano cheese or some roasted tofu. If not, you can serve with a lean pork chop or chicken breast.

Coconut Curry Tofu Bowl

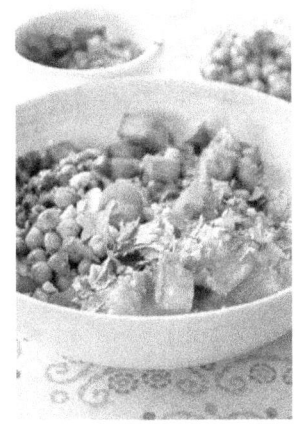

- Prep time: 15 minutes + 30 minutes
- Cooking time: 30 minutes
- Serving: 6
- Calories: 219kcal
- Fats: 8g|Carbs: 21g|Protein: 15g

INGREDIENTS

1. Grated ginger (1 tablespoon)
2. Extra-firm tofu (1 package)
3. Finely chopped seeded jalapeño pepper (1 medium)
4. Curry powder (2 tablespoons)
5. Coconut oil (3 teaspoons)
6. Chopped orange or yellow bell pepper (1 medium)
7. Minced garlic (4 teaspoons)
8. Chopped carrots (2 mediums)

9. Cumin powder (½ teaspoon)
Coconut milk, unflavored and unsweetened (2 cups)

Bok choy with the leaves and stems chopped (1 medium)

Cinnamon powder (⅛ teaspoon)

Canned tomato sauce (4 ounces)

10. Cauliflower rice
Low sodium chicken or vegetable stock (½ cup)

Finely chopped cilantro (¼ cup)

INSTRUCTIONS

1. Remove excess water from the tofu and place it in a bowl lined with paper towels. Place some extra layers of paper towel on top of the tofu. If you don't have extra paper towels, use a clean dish towel.
2. Place a heavy skillet on top of the paper towel or dish towel for extra weight. Leave that set up alone for about 30 minutes to drain as much water as possible.
3. Now transfer the tofu to a clean chopping board and slice it in half horizontally then dice it into 1-by-2- inch pieces. Set aside.
4. Place a large skillet over medium heat and drizzle 1 ½ teaspoons of coconut oil into it. As soon as the oil is hot and steaming, gently drop the tofu cubes into it to cook for about 15 minutes or until it looks golden brown on both sides. When it's ready, pour the tofu cubes into a dish and set aside.
5. Drizzle the leftover coconut oil, about 1 ½ teaspoons into the same pan used to fry the tofu. When the oil is hot and steaming, gently pour in ginger, bell pepper, bok choy stems,

jalapeño, garlic and carrots. Gently stir fry for 10 minutes or extra if the veggies are not tender enough.
6. Sprinkle turmeric powder, cinnamon powder, curry powder and cumin powder. Stir thoroughly.
7. Next thing to do is add tomato sauce, stock and coconut milk. Stir thoroughly
8. Add bok choy leaves and tofu then fold them in. Leave this to simmer for about 10 minutes or more if the leaves haven't wilted.
9. To serve, scoop some cauliflower rice into a bowl then top with tofu sauce. For garnishing, use cilantro.

Notes: This recipe can be used as a base for other versions of it so don't be afraid to change it up. Swap some veggies for another like spinach or kale in place of bok choy, carrots in place of sweet potatoes, etc. Throw in some butternut squash and other frozen mixed vegetables. Keep in mind that it is easier to use vegetables that are in season.

Curried Eggplant And Chickpea Quinoa

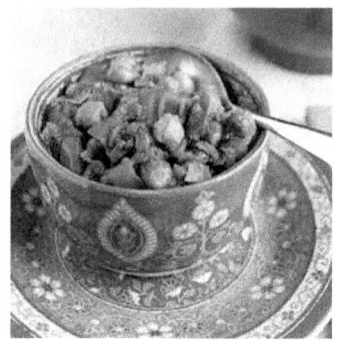

- Prep time: 15 minutes
- Cooking time: 20 minutes
- Serving: 8
- Calories: 131kcal
- Fats: 2g|Carbs: 23g|Protein: 6g

INGREDIENTS

1. Diced red bell pepper (1 medium)
2. Cayenne pepper (¼ teaspoon)
3. Extra virgin olive oil (1 teaspoon)
4. Smoked paprika (2 teaspoons)
5. Minced garlic (4 teaspoons)
6. Chopped onion (1 large)
7. Water (½ cup)
8. Turmeric powder (1 teaspoon)
9. Chicken and vegetable stock (1 cup)

Chopped eggplant (1 medium)

Chopped tomatoes (3 medium)

Low-fat plain Greek yogurt

Drained and rinsed chickpeas (1 can)

Chopped yellow summer squash (1 medium)

Packaged quinoa (½ cup)

INSTRUCTIONS

1. Drizzle olive oil into a large pan and place it over medium heat. Pour in garlic and stir fry for about 1 minute. Stir in bell pepper and onion, then continue to stir fry for about 3 minutes or until soft.
2. Sprinkle turmeric, cayenne pepper, cumin and smoked paprika. Leave to cook for 2 minutes.
3. Stir in eggplant, tomatoes, chickpeas, squash and water. Place a lid on the pan and lower the heat just a little bit and let it cook for 15 minutes.
4. Meanwhile, as you wait for the chickpeas and veggies to cook, whip about a saucepan and place it over medium heat. In goes the stock and quinoa. Cover the saucepan and leave it to boil. Once that happens, lower the heat and allow it to simmer until the quinoa absorbs all the stock. This usually takes about 15 minutes.
5. Take the saucepan off the heat and fluff the quinoa.
6. To serve, scoop some quinoa into a plate and serve with curried vegetables and a scoop of yogurt.

Notes: Be careful when selecting your high-protein grains. Ancient grains are the most protein-rich in the game. Quinoa, barley, amaranth and millet will not let you down. Doubt me? Next time you go grocery shopping, take a peek at the label on your whole grains.

Chapter 8: Seafood Recipes

Tuna Noodle-Less Casserole

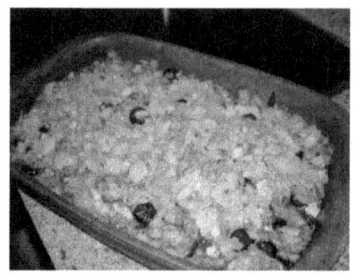

- Prep time: 15 minutes
- Cooking time: 40 minutes
- Serving: 10
- Calories: 147kcal
- Fats: 7g|Carbs: 6g|Protein: 15g

INGREDIENTS

1. Diced bell pepper (1 medium)
2. Olive oil-based mayonnaise (⅓ cup)
3. Low-fat milk (½ cup)
4. Diced red onion (1 medium)
5. Fresh green beans (3 cups)
6. Grated cheddar cheese (1 cup)
7. Chopped tomato (1 ½ cups)
8. Black pepper powder (½ teaspoon)

9. Condensed cream of mushroom soup (1 can)
Nonstick cooking spray

Water-packed albacore tuna (8 cans)

INSTRUCTIONS

1. Prepare your oven. Preheat to 425°F.
2. Grease a large pan with cooking spray and set it over medium heat. Pour in red bell pepper, tomatoes and onion then stir fry for 5 minutes or more if the tomatoes haven't softened yet. Take the pan off the heat.
3. Remove the stem ends of your green beans and snap beans into 3-inch bits.
4. Now pour water into a pot, enough to fill a third of it and set a steamer basket inside. Set the pot over high heat until the water starts to boil.
5. Pour the green beans into the steamer basket and cover the pot. Lower the heat so that the green beans will steam for 5 minutes. Once that is done, remove the basket, drain the water and set the green beans aside.
6. Grease a baking dish with cooking spray.
7. Pour cheese, mayonnaise, milk and condensed soup into a large bowl and mix thoroughly. Sprinkle black pepper over the mixture and mix again.
8. Pour green beans, stir fried veggies and tuna into the mayonnaise mixture and stir gently to mix. Transfer the mixture to the greased baking dish and place it in the oven to bake until you notice brown edges. About 30 minutes.
9. Serve warm.

Notes: Modifying this recipe is super easy. If you want to give its protein content a boost, here's what you need to do. Use ½ cup of nonfat cheese and slash the mayonnaise by 2 tablespoons. If you want a nice puree, use an immersion blender. If you want a slightly different flavor, you will have to stir fry the chopped tomatoes first in a pan coated with 1 teaspoon of olive oil. Stir fry for 5 minutes before adding the remaining vegetables.

Herb-Crusted Salmon

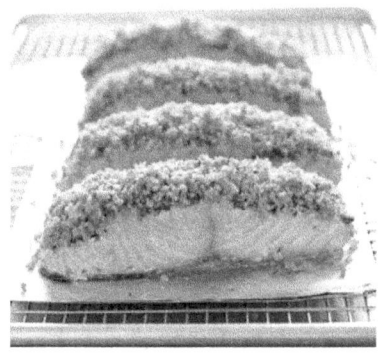

- Prep time: 10 minutes
- Cooking: 20 minutes
- Serving: 2
- Calories: 197kcal
- Fats: 10g|Carbs: 9g|Protein: 27g

INGREDIENTS

1. Minced garlic (2 teaspoons)
2. Dried thyme (½ teaspoon)

3. Shredded Parmigiano-Reggiano cheese (4 tablespoons)
4. Salmon fillets (2 medium)
5. Fresh lemon juice (2 teaspoons)
6. Dried parsley (1 tablespoon)

INSTRUCTIONS

1. Prepare your oven. Preheat to 425°F.
2. Prepare a sheet pan. Line it with parchment paper.
3. Get your salmon and place it on the parchment lined sheet pan then cover with another layer of parchment paper. Place this in the oven to bake for roughly 10 minutes.
4. While the salmon is baking, pour lemon juice, garlic, Parmigiano-Reggiano cheese, parsley and thyme into a small bowl. Mix thoroughly and set aside.
5. Bring out the sheet pan and discard parchment paper on top of the salmon. Using a pastry brush glaze the salmon with the garlic mixture and place it back in the oven to bake for an additional 5 minutes. No need to cover it with another piece of parchment paper.
6. You'll know the fish is ready when you can flake it easily using a fork. Serve warm.

Notes: Avoid overcooking the salmon because it will turn rubbery and that fishy flavor will just go from zero to a hundred. To be extra safe, use a meat thermometer. The internal temperature of a properly cooked fish should read 145°F.

Slow-Roasted Pesto Salmon

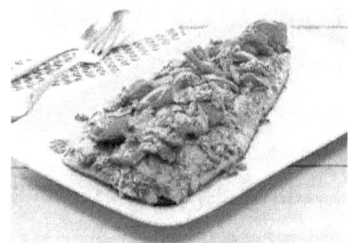

- Prep time: 5 minutes
- Cooking time: 20 minutes
- Serving: 4
- Calories: 180kcal
- Fats: 10g|Carbs: 1g|Protein: 20g

INGREDIENTS

1. Extra virgin olive oil (1 teaspoon)
2. Salmon fillets (4 medium)
3. Perfect basil pesto (4 tablespoons)

INSTRUCTIONS

1. Prepare your oven. Preheat to 275°F.
2. Using aluminum foil, line a rimmed sheet pan and then coat the foil with olive oil.
3. Arrange the salmon fillets in the sheet pan with the skin side down
4. Pour 1 tablespoon of pesto on top of the salmon fillets and place sheet pan in the oven to bake until the center looks opaque. This usually takes 20 minutes.

5. Serve immediately.

Lemon-Parsley Crab Cakes

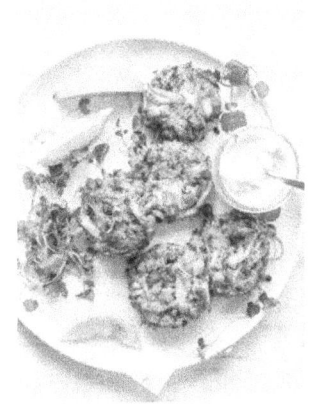

- Prep time: 15 minutes + 30 minutes
- Cooking time: 10 minutes
- Serving: 4
- Calories: 148kcal
- Fats: 4g | Carbs: 5g | Protein: 21g

INGREDIENTS

1. Lightly beaten egg (1 large)
2. Cayenne pepper powder (¼ teaspoon)

3. Whole wheat bread crumbs (3 tablespoons)
4. Finely chopped parsley (2 teaspoons)
5. Dijon mustard (½ teaspoon)
6. Olive oil-based mayonnaise (1 ½ tablespoons)
7. Drained lump crab meat with the cartilage removed (2 cans)
8. Fresh lemon juice (½ lemon)
9. Nonstick cooking spray

INSTRUCTIONS

1. Pour breadcrumbs, mayonnaise, egg, lemon juice, cayenne pepper, mustard and parsley into a medium sized bowl. Mix thoroughly.
2. Pour the lump crabmeat into the bowl and gently fold it into the mixture.
3. Use a ¼-cup measuring cup to mold the mixture into four patties. Place the individual patties in the fridge to stand for 30 minutes.
4. Prepare your oven while the patties get ready. Heat to 500°F. Grease a sheet pan with enough cooking spray and set aside.
5. When the crab cakes are ready, place them on the sheet pan and slide them into the oven to bake for 10 minutes. Keep it at the center rack of the oven for even heat distribution.
6. Serve warm.

Notes: If you walk into a restaurant to grab a crab cake, you'll most likely be hit with the crumb-filled-oil-fried ones. They might taste great but now it's all about healthy eating, right? Opt for broiled, baked or grilled seafood instead if you must have something at the restaurant.

Seafood Cioppino

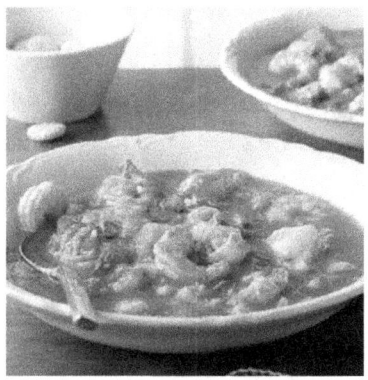

- Prep time: 25 minutes
- Cooking time: 35 minutes
- Serving: 8
- Calories: 171kcal
- Fats: 4g | Carbs: 5g | Protein: 21g

INGREDIENTS

1. Dry white wine (1 ½ cups)
2. Minced garlic (2 teaspoons)
3. Water (4 cups)
4. Extra virgin olive oil (1 tablespoon)
5. Grape tomatoes (1 container)
6. Chopped green bell pepper (1 medium)
7. Sliced whole leeks (2 medium)
8. Dried thyme (½ teaspoon)
9. Chopped (2 stalks)

Dried basil (½ teaspoon)

Finely chopped parsley (1 tablespoon)

Chopped tomato (1 large)

Deveined shrimp (2 pounds)

Black pepper powder (1 teaspoon)

10. Bay leaf (1 leaf)
Drained crab mean with the cartilage removed (1 can)

Fresh lemon juice (½ lemon)

11. Scallops (½ pound)

INSTRUCTIONS

1. If you have a Dutch oven, awesome. If not, you can use a large pot. Place wuther over medium heat. Drizzle in olive oil and pour in garlic. Stir fry the garlic for about 2 minutes then pour in leeks and stir some more for an additional 2 minutes or until soft.
2. Stir in green pepper and celery. Leave to cook for roughly 5 minutes or extra if it isn't tender enough.
3. Time to add water, tomatoes, bay leaf, wine, thyme, lemon juice, basil and parsley. Stir and leave to boil.
4. Lower the heat and leave the mixture to simmer for about 25 minutes.
5. Use a spoon to take out and dispose of the bay leaf then add crab meat, scallops and shrimp. Let that simmer for 10 minutes or until the shrimp loses its pink tinge and the scallops look a bit opaque.
6. Sprinkle in black pepper powder and stir.
7. Serve in soup bowls. Enjoy

Notes: If you would like a little variety in this recipe, you can throw in some white fish or fresh mussels. Homemade croutons from whole wheat bread will totally go with this recipe if you are into that sort of thing.

Chapter 9: Poultry Recipes

Slow Cooker White Chicken Chili

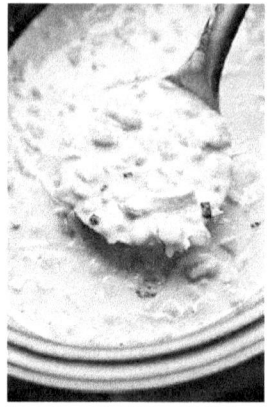

- Prep time: 10 minutes
- Cooking time: 6 hours
- Serving: 6
- Calories: 225kcal
- Fats: 3g|Carbs: 25g|Protein: 26g

INGREDIENTS

1. Chopped onion (1 large)
2. Ground coriander (1 ½ teaspoons)
3. Drained and rinsed chickpeas (2 cans)
4. Minced seedless jalapeño pepper (1 medium)
5. Chili powder (2 teaspoons)

6. Low sodium chicken stock (2 cups)
7. Cumin powder (1 tablespoon)
8. Chicken breasts with the skin and bone removed (1 pound)
9. Chopped green chiles (1 can)

Dried oregano (2 teaspoons)

Freshly chopped cilantro (¼ cup)

10. Water (2 cups)

INSTRUCTIONS

1. You will be making the bean puree first. Pour 1 can of beans into a blender and add 1 cup of stock. Pulse on high until smooth and set aside.
2. Toss the chicken breasts into a slow cooker and season with coriander, chili powder, onion, cumin, oregano, green chiles and jalapeños.
3. Stir in whatever stock and beans you have left then add water and the bean puree.
4. Place a lid on the cooker and lower the heat. This should cook for 6 hours so you can either set the timer or use an alarm clock.
5. When 5 ½ hours are up, place the chicken on a tray and shred it with two forks. When that is done, pour it back into the slow cooker and let it cook still on low heat for an extra 25 minutes or until the chicken absorbs quite a bit of the sauce.
6. Serve in soup bowls and top with cilantro. Enjoy!

Notes: Spicy foods are believed to assist with weight loss because after having a meal with that extra spicy tinge, you will notice that you might not want to eat as much as you normally would have. The argument about the ability of spicy peppers to quicken metabolism is still on so there isn't a verdict yet. But I know for sure that you won't rush your food if it has added peppers like some additional jalapeño. Another plus, jalapeños are absolutely filled with antioxidants.

Grilled Chicken Wings

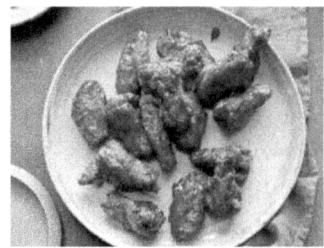

- Prep time: 15 minutes
- Cooking time: 20 minutes
- Serving: 18
- Calories: 82kcal
- Fats: 6g|Carbs: 1g|Protein: 7g

INGREDIENTS

1. Garlic powder (1 teaspoon)
2. Extra virgin olive oil (1 teaspoon)
3. Black pepper powder (1 teaspoon)
4. Buffalo wing sauce like Frank's red-hot (1 cup)
5. Frozen chicken wings (1½ pounds)

INSTRUCTIONS

1. I hope you have a grill! Heat it to 350°F.
2. Sprinkle both sides of chicken wings with garlic powder and black pepper powder.
3. Place the wings on the grill to roast for 30 minutes. Each side gets 15 minutes. If done right, both sides will look crisp and golden brown.
4. Place the wings in a bowl of buffalo wing sauce plus olive oil and toss to coat.
5. Serve warm.

Notes: Avoid the skin as often as you can. Just go straight for the meat. During the first few days or weeks post op, a lot of people are unable to stomach skin on turkey or chicken because of its density. However, after about 9 months post-op, you might be able to tolerate maybe 1 or 2 deep fried skin on turkey, but portions must be limited due to the amount of fat contained in skin. If wings happen to be your favorite, you can make yourself happy with this recipe.

Ranch-Seasoned Crispy Chicken Tenders

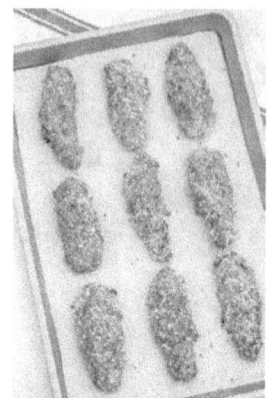

- Prep time: 10 minutes
- Cooking time: 20 minutes
- Serving: 6
- Calories: 162kcal
- Fats: 2g|Carbs: 8g|Protein: 25g

INGREDIENTS

1. Lightly beaten egg (1 egg)
2. Shredded Parmigiano-Reggiano cheese (2 tablespoons)
3. Chicken tenderloin (6 pieces)
4. Dried dill (¾ teaspoon)
5. Dried basil (¼ teaspoon)
6. Dried parsley (2 teaspoons)
7. Onion powder (¼ teaspoon)
8. Black pepper powder (⅛ teaspoon)
9. Whole wheat bread crumbs (½ cup)

Nonstick cooking spray

Garlic powder (¼ teaspoon)

Whole wheat pastry flour (2 tablespoons)

INSTRUCTIONS

1. Prepare your oven. Heat to 425°F.
2. Coat a sheet pan with nonstick cooking spray.
3. Whip about three small bowls. Put flour in one, lightly beaten egg in another and a mixture of Parmigiano-Reggiano cheese, garlic powder, parsley, bread crumbs, dill, basil, black pepper powder and onion powder in the last one
4. You're going to dip the tenderloins one at a time into all the bowls starting with the flour and shaking off the excess then moving on to the egg and finally the breadcrumbs mixture. Toss it around in it to thoroughly coat.
5. Place the coated tenderloin on the sheet pan and repeat step 4 until all the tenderloins are coated. Place the sheet pan in the oven and bake for roughly 25 minutes so it properly browns and cooks through.
6. Serve warm.

Notes: This recipe can be transformed into a buffalo ranch chicken salad as easy as ABC. All you will need to do is coat the tenderloins in Frank's red-hot buffalo wing sauce and dice them into bite-sized bits. Throw them into a bowl of shredded carrots, tomatoes, and mixed greens. Scoop low fat blue cheese into the mixture and drizzle it with creamy peppercorn ranch dressing. Voila! It's a salad.

Chicken "Nachos" With Sweet Bell Peppers

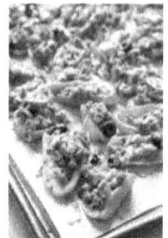

- Prep time: 10 minutes
- Cooking time: 25 minutes
- Serving: 16
- Calories: 189kcal
- Fats: 3g|Carbs: 29g|Protein: 9g

INGREDIENTS

1. Minced onion (½ medium)
2. Cumin powder (1 teaspoon)
3. Halved seeded mini bell peppers (1 package)
4. Diced tomato (1 large)
5. Extra virgin olive oil (2 teaspoons)
6. Smoked paprika (½ teaspoon)
7. Cooked shredded chicken breast (2 cups)
8. Grated Colby jack cheese (1 cup)
9. Nonstick cooking spray

Finely chopped scallions (3 medium)

Garlic powder (1 teaspoon)

Thinly sliced seedless jalapeño pepper (1 medium)

Chopped black olives (¼ cup)

INSTRUCTIONS

1. Prepare your oven, heat to 400°F.
2. Prepare a sheet pan by lining it with aluminum foil. Now generously grease the foil with cooking spray.
3. Place the bell pepper halves with the skin side down on the sheet pan. Set aside
4. Pour olive oil into a large pan and set it over medium heat. Pour in the onion and stir fry for about 2 minutes. Now throw in the chicken, garlic powder, smoked paprika, tomato, and cumin. Stir and leave to cook for roughly 5 minutes or until the chicken is thoroughly cooked and the tomato looks soft enough.
5. Now scoop a full tablespoon of the chicken mixture into a bell pepper cup. Layer with cheese, scallions, jalapeño and black olives. Repeat this process until all the bell pepper cups are filled.
6. Slide sheet pan into the oven to bake until the cheese completely melts. This should take 15 minutes.
7. Serve warm.

Notes: If you don't have the energy to rush to the grocery store, you can always shred any leftover chicken you have. You can also just purchase a rotisserie chicken and shred that. If you want to transform this recipe into a whole meal, just serve with refried black beans and avocado slice toppings.

Baked "Fried Chicken" Thighs

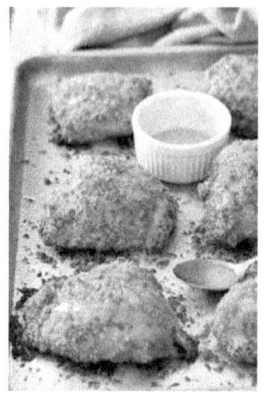

- Prep time: 10 minutes
- Cooking time: 35 minutes
- Serving: 4
- Calories: 272kcal
- Fats: 8g|Carbs: 15g|Protein: 25g

INGREDIENTS

1. Eggs (2 large)
2. Smoked paprika (1 teaspoon)
3. Cayenne pepper (½ teaspoon)
4. Garlic powder (½ teaspoons)
5. Water (1 tablespoon)
6. Black pepper powder (½ teaspoon)
7. Dried oregano (½ teaspoon)
8. Dijon mustard (1 teaspoon)
9. Nonstick cooking spray

Bran flakes (2 ½ cups)

Skinned boneless chicken thighs (4 medium)

INSTRUCTIONS

1. Prepare your oven. Heat to 400°F.
2. Get an aluminum-lined sheet pan ready and slide it into the oven underneath a clean oven rack. Grease the oven rack with cooking spray.
3. Get a large zip lock bag and pour in smoked paprika, cayenne pepper, garlic powder, oregano and black pepper powder. Toss the chicken thighs into the bag and seal it. Squeeze the bag and contents to coat the chicken with seasoning. Leave it alone for a minute.
4. Mix mustard, eggs and water in a small dish until thoroughly combined. Set aside.
5. Pour the bran flakes into another zip lock bag and squeeze to crush it.
6. Now for the chicken, bring out a seasoned chicken thigh and dip it in the mustard mixture and then into the bag of crushed bran flakes. Squeeze the bag to coat and place the thigh on the coated oven rack. Repeat the process until all the chicken thighs have been breaded.
7. If you're wondering why the thighs aren't going into the sheet pan, it is because the sheet pan is just there to catch any liquid that may drip from the chicken thighs above it.
8. Let the chicken bake in the oven until the thighs look crisp. This takes 35 minutes or less.
9. Serve warm.

Notes: White meat chicken is a little lower in saturated fat content than the dark meat counterpart but dark meat is usually more tender and moister than chicken breast, so don't be afraid to indulge, especially after surgery when you will need foods with a soft texture. This meal goes well with cheesy cauliflower casserole and any veggies you might like to add.

Chapter 10: Snacks And Dessert

Superfood Dark Chocolates

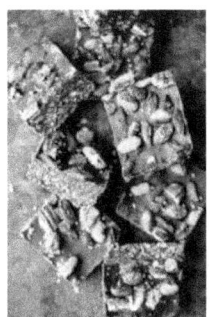

- Prep time: 5 minutes
- Cooking time: 25 minutes
- Serving: 18
- Calories: 102kcal
- Fats: 7g | Carbs: 8g | Protein: 3g

INGREDIENTS

1. Chopped pumpkin seeds (¼ cup)
2. Unsweetened grated coconut (¼ cup)
3. Sea salt (1 teaspoon)
4. Chopped pecans (¼ cup)
5. Dark chocolate chips like Ghirardelli dark chocolate chips (6 ounces)
6. Unsweetened dried wild blueberries (¼ cup)

INSTRUCTIONS

1. Prepare two sheet pans. Line them with parchment paper.
2. Pour water into a pot, enough to fill it. Leave it to boil. Once it boils, lower the heat and put a stainless steel bowl in the pot so it floats on top of the water
3. Pour the chocolate chips into the steel bowl and stir until it melts completely. If this method seems too complicated for you, you can always put the chocolate chips in a microwave-safe bowl and melt it in the microwave.
4. Drizzle the liquid chocolate onto the sheet pan in squares and pour in some pumpkin seeds, pecans, dried blueberries, coconut and any other thing you'd like in your superfood into each square. Sprinkle sea salt over all the squares and place it in the fridge to harden.
5. To preserve, put the chocolate squares in an airtight bowl and store them in the fridge. It will keep for only two weeks.

Notes: You should change up your chocolate toppings every now and then. Chia seeds will give you some fiber and extra crunch. Other dried fruits like cranberries, mango and sliced figs. You can also substitute the other nuts in the recipe for shelled pistachios and cashews. Don't forget, control your portions because dried fruits have a high sugar and calorie content.

Chocolate Chia Pudding

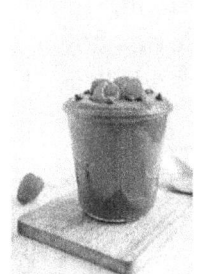

- Prep time: 15 minutes + 1 hour
- Cooking time: 0 minutes
- Serving: 4
- Calories: 182kcal
- Fats: 9g|Carbs: 14g|Protein: 11g

INGREDIENTS

1. Liquid stevia (10 drops)
2. Fresh raspberries ⅟1/2 cup)
3. Unsweetened soy milk (2 cups)
4. Vanilla extract (¼ teaspoon)
5. Chia seeds (½ cup)
6. Cinnamon powder (¼ teaspoon)
7. Cocoa powder, unsweetened (¼ teaspoon)

INSTRUCTIONS

1. Mix cinnamon powder, soy milk, cocoa powder, vanilla extract and stevia in a small bowl until they are thoroughly mixed.
2. Pour in chia seeds and stir again.
3. Scoop into four small serving bowls.
4. Put lids on the bowls and place them in the fridge for an hour so it will set.
5. Top with raspberries when ready to eat!

Chocolate Brownies With Almond Butter

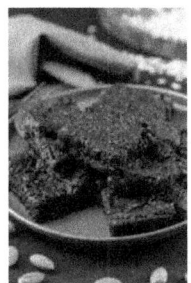

- Prep time: 5 minutes
- Cooking time: 25 minutes
- Serving: 16
- Calories: 124kcal
- Fats: 9g|Carbs: 11g|Protein: 3g

INGREDIENTS

1. Ground flaxseed (1 tablespoon)
2. Vanilla extract (1 teaspoon)
3. Cocoa powder (½ cup)
4. Almond butter (½ cup)
5. Agave nectar (½ cup)
6. Baking soda (¼ teaspoon)
7. Eggs (2 large)
8. Nonstick cooking spray
9. Melted coconut oil (¼ cup)

Instant coffee powder (½ teaspoon)

INSTRUCTIONS

1. Prepare your oven. Heat to 325°F.
2. Grease a glass baking dish with nonstick cooking spray.
3. Pour the baking soda, instant powder, almond butter, flaxseed, agave nectar, eggs, cocoa powder, coconut oil and eggs into a blender. Pulse on high until you get a smooth mixture then transfer the batter into greased baking dish.
4. Slide the dish into the oven and bake for about 25 minutes or until you poke the middle with a knife and it comes out clean.
5. Set it aside to cool for about 10 minutes before slicing it into squares.

Notes: Don't forget, portion control is everything. Don't overindulge. Store the brownies in small portions in Ziplock bags. Leave them to thaw out properly before serving.

Lemon-Blackberry Frozen Yogurt

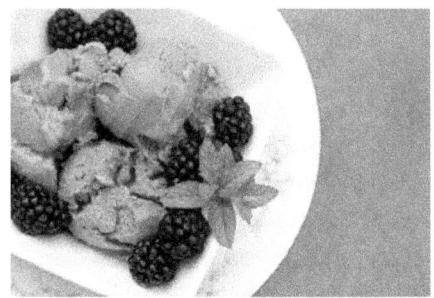

- Prep time: 10 minutes
- Cooking time: 0 minutes
- Serving: 4
- Calories: 68kcal
- Fats: 0g|Carbs: 15g|Protein: 3g

INGREDIENTS

1. Fresh lemon juice (1 lemon)
2. Frozen blackberries (4 cups)
3. Liquid stevia (2 teaspoons)
4. Low fat plain Greek yogurt (½ cup)
5. Fresh mint leaves for toppings

INSTRUCTIONS

1. Throw the blackberries into a blender. Scoop in some yogurt. Pour in stevia and lemon juice. Pulse on high until you get a smooth mixture. This should take 5 minutes or less.

2. You can choose to serve right away or store it in an airtight bowl. Store in the fridge for 3 weeks. For toppings, go with mint leaves.

Notes: Jazz up your fro-yo. Get creative with the flavors. Make use of low sugar flavored Greek yogurt sometimes and try out herbs if you'd like. Watermelon with cayenne pepper and lime or mango and coconut.

Old-Fashioned Apple Crisp

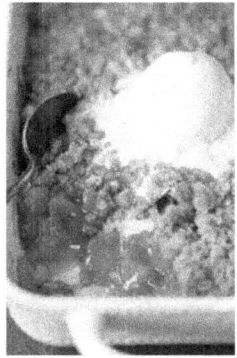

- Prep time: 15 minutes
- Cooking time: 45 minutes
- Serving: 10
- Calories: 170kcal
- Fats: 6g | Carbs: 28g | Protein: 3g

INGREDIENTS

1. Stevia powder (3 teaspoons)
2. Chopped cored skinless apples (6 medium)
3. Cinnamon powder (½ teaspoons)
4. Water (½ cup)
5. Fresh lemon juice (½ lemon)
6. Old fashioned oats (¾ cup)
7. Cornstarch (1 tablespoon)
8. Whole wheat pastry flour (¾ cup)
9. Nutmeg powder (¼ teaspoon)
   Low-fat plain yogurt (½ cup)

Nonstick cooking spray

Melted coconut oil (¼ cup)

INSTRUCTIONS

1. Prepare your oven. Heat to 350°F.
2. Grease a baking dish with nonstick cooking spray.
3. Pour water into the dish. Stir in apples, cinnamon powder, 1 ½ teaspoons of stevia, nutmeg powder, lemon juice and cornstarch. Slide the dish into the oven to bake for about 20 minutes.
4. While that is happening, mix flour, leftover stevia and oats in a smaller bowl. Add coconut oil and yogurt. Stir until it is thoroughly mixed and moist.
5. Bring out the baking dish and pour the oatmeal mixture all over the mixture then slide it back into the oven to bake for an additional 25 minutes.
6. Serve warm.

Notes: Ever tried grilling or baking your fruits? This will boost its natural flavor. If you can get your hands on some alternative version of fruit crisp of some fruits like pears, cherries and peaches.

No-Bake Peanut Butter Protein Bites With Dark Chocolate

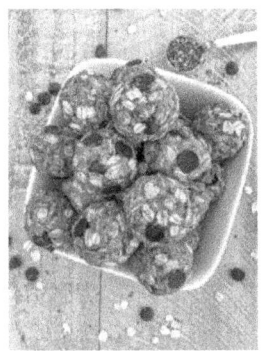

- Prep time: 20 minutes + 30 minutes
- Cooking time: 0 minutes
- Serving: 25
- Calories: 181kcal
- Fats: 10g|Carbs: 11g|Protein: 11g

INGREDIENTS

1. Vanilla protein powder (1 cup)
2. Vanilla extract (1 teaspoon)
3. Ground flaxseed (2 tablespoons)
4. Old fashioned rolled oats (1 cup)
5. Dark chocolate chips (¼ cup)
6. Smooth 100% natural peanut butter (¾ cup)
7. Chia seeds (1 tablespoon)
8. Water (As much as you need)
9. Stevia baking blend (¾ teaspoon)

INSTRUCTIONS

1. Pour flaxseed, vanilla extract, protein powder, chia seeds, peanut butter, oats, water, chocolate chips and stevia into a large bowl. Mix thoroughly.
2. Place the bowl in the refrigerator for about 30 minutes or until it hardens a bit.
3. Make 25 balls out of the mixture and serve immediately
4. To store, put in an airtight container. If you want it to keep for longer than a week, store it in the freezer.

Notes: Cooking tip: Mix and match the dry or wet ingredients to make simple

swaps. Add coconut and cocoa powder for a chocolate fix, or try sunflower

seed butter instead of peanut butter to go nut-free. You can also add some

pumpkin puree and cinnamon for a fall treat.

Chapter 11: Sauces And Seasoning

Greek Salad Dressing

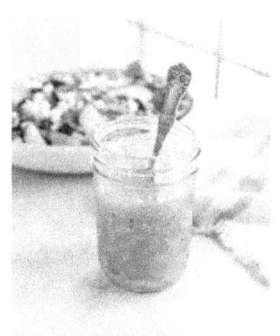

- Prep time: 10 minutes
- Cooking time: 0 minutes
- Serving: 1
- Calories: 89kcal
- Fats: 9g|Carbs: 1g|Protein: 0g

INGREDIENTS

1. Dried basil (1 teaspoon)
2. Extra virgin olive oil (⅓ cup)
3. Dijon mustard (½ teaspoon)
4. Fresh lemon juice (1 lemon)
5. Red wine vinegar (½ cup)
6. Minced garlic (4 teaspoons)

7. Black pepper powder (½ teaspoon)
8. Dried oregano (1 tablespoon)

INSTRUCTIONS

1. Mix olive oil, oregano, pepper, garlic, mustard, basil and lemon juice in a medium sized bowl. Another way to do this is to pour all the ingredients into a mason jar and shake thoroughly until it's all mixed up.
2. Stir in the red wine vinegar and that's done,
3. You can choose to serve immediately or store it in an airtight bowl and place it in the refrigerator. Whenever you want to use it, leave it to sit for 15 minutes for it to defrost. Stir thoroughly right before use.

Notes: You can jazz up your salad by substituting your usual iceberg lettuce salad for a Mediterranean Greek salad.

Creamy Peppercorn Ranch Dressing

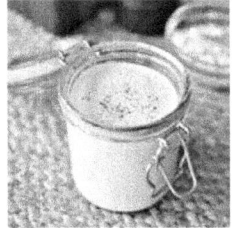

- Prep time: 10 minutes
- Cooking time: 0 minutes
- Serving: 1 cup
- Calories: 35kcal
- Fat: 1g | Carbs: 2g | Protein: 4g

INGREDIENTS

1. Onion flakes (½ teaspoon)
2. Low fat plain Greek yogurt (¾ cup)
3. Shredded Parmigiano-Reggiano cheese (⅓ cup)
4. Fresh lemon juice (1 lemon)
5. Salt (¼ teaspoon)
6. Low fat buttermilk (¼ cup)
7. Black pepper powder (2 teaspoons)

INSTRUCTIONS

1. Pour the yogurt, buttermilk, onion flakes, lemon juice, salt and pepper into a blender and pulse on high until you get a creamy and smooth mixture.

Notes: This dressing goes well with raw veggies. It can also serve as a condiment for a turkey wrap or as a garnish for a turkey burger.

Mango Salsa

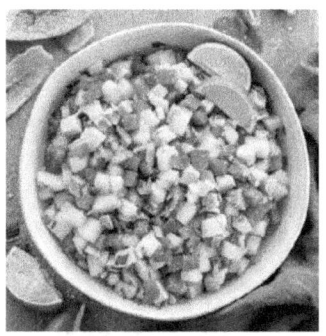

- Prep time: 15 minutes
- Cooking time: 0 minutes
- Serving: 2
- Calories: 27kcal
- Fats: 0g | Carbs: 7g | Protein: 0g

INGREDIENTS

1. Freshly squeezed lime juice (2 limes)
2. Skinned and chopped mango (1 large)
3. Finely chopped red onion (¼ cup)
4. Chopped fresh cilantro (¼ cup)
5. Chopped seedless jalapeños (1 medium)

INSTRUCTIONS

1. Get a medium sized bowl. Pour in mango, lime juice, onion, cilantro and jalapeño. That's it!
2. Serve immediately or store in an airtight bowl and place in the fridge.

Perfect Basil Pesto

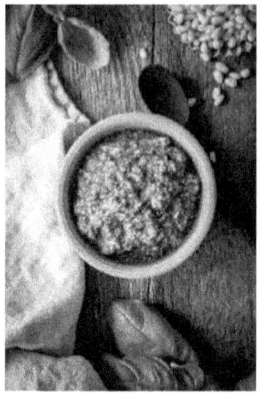

- Prep time: 5 minutes
- Cooking time: 0 minutes
- Serving: 5
- Calories: 99kcal
- Fats: 10g|Carbs: 1g|Protein: 2g

INGREDIENTS

1. Parmigiano-Reggiano cheese (¼ cup)
2. Pine nuts (2 tablespoons)
3. Fresh basil leaves (1 cup)
4. Water (2 tablespoons)
5. Extra virgin olive oil (2 ½ tablespoons)

INSTRUCTION

1. Pour Parmigiano-Reggiano cheese, pine nuts, basil, water and olive oil into a blender and pulse on high until you get a smooth mixture.
2. You can choose to serve right away or store it in an airtight bowl in the refrigerator.

Notes: I won't lie, pine nuts are a bit expensive, so if you can't afford them, just use an equal amount of almonds or walnuts. They will work just fine.

Marinara Sauce With Italian Herbs

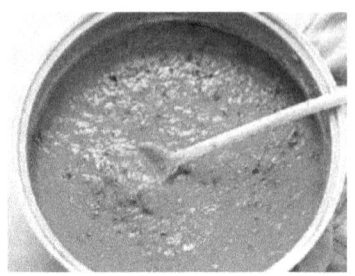

- Prep time: 5 minutes
- Cooking time: 35 minutes
- Serving: 3
- Calories: 37kcal
- Fats: 0g|Carbs: 7g|Protein: 0g

INGREDIENTS

1. Dried oregano (1 teaspoon)
2. Extra virgin olive oil (1 teaspoon)
3. Dried basil (1 teaspoon)
4. Minced garlic (1 teaspoon)
5. Diced whole tomatoes (12 medium)
6. Diced yellow onion (½ large)
7. Red pepper flakes (¼ teaspoon)
8. Finely chopped red bell pepper †1 medium)
9. Bay leaves (2 leaves)

INSTRUCTIONS

1. Set a saucepan over medium heat. Drizzle olive oil into it and stir fry the garlic for about 1 minute.
2. Stir in red bell pepper and onion then leave to cook for about 2 minutes. Don't forget to stir in between.
3. Now pour in red pepper flakes, tomatoes, basil and oregano. Stir carefully to mix.
4. Throw the bay leaves into the mix then cover and lower the heat so it simmers for 30 minutes.
5. Once 30 minutes is up, take off the lid and dispose of the bay leaves.
6. To puree the mixture, make use of an immersion blender if you have one or just use a blender.
7. Serve warm.

Notes: This recipe can be used as a condiment to spice up the bland foods during the puree stage. To change it up, blend with ground beef or stir in some cottage or ricotta cheese.

Chapter 12: Soups And Salads

Creamy Chicken Soup With Cauliflower

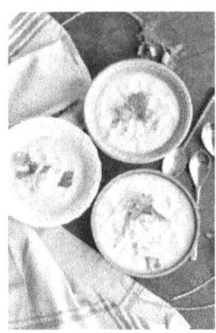

- Prep time: 15 minutes
- Cooking time: 40 minutes
- Serving: 8
- Calories: 164kcal
- Fats: 3g| Carbs: 5g|Protein: 25g

INGREDIENTS

1. Diced yellow onion (½ medium)
2. Chopped cooked chicken breast (4 medium)
3. Minced garlic (1 teaspoon)
4. Dried thyme (1 teaspoon)
5. Diced celery (1 stalk)
6. Water (2 cups)

7. Extra virgin olive oil (1 teaspoon)
8. Low Sodium chicken stock (2 cups)
9. Chopped carrot (1 medium)

Cauliflower florets (2 ½ cups)

Black pepper powder (1 teaspoon)

Nonfat milk (2 cups)

Chopped fresh spinach (1 cup)

INSTRUCTIONS

1. Set a large pot over medium heat. Drizzle in olive oil and stir fry the garlic for just 1 minute. Pour in carrot, celery and onion then stir fry again for about 5 minutes.
2. Throw in chicken breast. Pour water and stock. Sprinkle black pepper, cauliflower and thyme. Lower the heat and let the mixture simmer uncovered for just 30 minutes.
3. Now throw in fresh spinach and cook for 5 minutes or more of the leaves don't look wilted.
4. Pour milk, stir and serve!

Baked Potato Soup

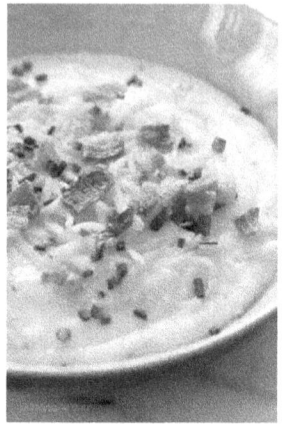

- Prep time: 10 minutes
- Cooking time: 30 minutes
- Serving: 6
- Calories: 181kcal
- Fats: 9g | Carbs: 18g | Protein: 9g

INGREDIENTS

1. Freshly chopped chives (4 tablespoons)
2. Whole wheat flour (3 tablespoons)
3. Low-fat plain Greek yogurt (½ cup)
4. Nitrate-free turkey bacon (4 slices)
5. Chicken or vegetable stock (1 ½ cups)
6. Grated sharp cheddar cheese (½ cup)
7. 1% milk (1 ½ cups)
8. Extra virgin olive oil (2 tablespoons)
9. Chopped russet potatoes (3 medium)

INSTRUCTIONS

1. Set a large pot over medium-high heat.
2. Throw in bacon and cook until both sides are crisp. This takes 10 minutes. Flip at the 5 minute mark. When it is cooked through, place it on a plate lined with paper towels to catch the excess oil. When it is cool enough to touch, cut it into fine cubes.
3. Drizzle olive oil into the same pot and stir in flour. Continue stirring for about 3 minutes or until it looks brown. Pour in the milk and stir continuously until it starts to look like a thick mixture. Now stir in the stock.
4. Throw in potatoes and leave to boil. Lower the heat and leave the soup to simmer until potatoes are soft enough to be pierced with a fork. This should take 20 minutes.
5. Scoop Greek yogurt into the mixture and stir.
6. Serve soup with cheese, turkey bacon, an extra scoop of yogurt and chives.

Notes: If you choose to have this during the puree stage post-op, add about 2 tablespoons of unflavored protein powder or egg white powder to ramp up the protein content.

Chicken, Barley, And Vegetable Soup

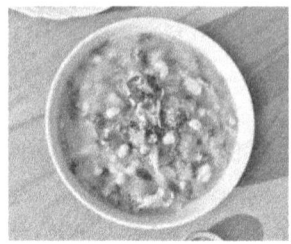

- Prep time: 15 minutes
- Cooking time: 50 minutes
- Serving: 8
- Calories: 198lcal
- Fats: 3g|Carbs: 9g|Protein: 16g

INGREDIENTS

1. Diced onion (1 large)
2. Pearl barley (¾ cup)
3. Chopped large carrots (2 large)
4. Extra virgin oil (1 tablespoon)
5. Chopped, cooked chicken (2 ½ cups)
6. Minced garlic (1 teaspoon)
7. Chopped celery (3 stalks)
8. Low sodium chicken broth (4 cups)
9. Diced tomatoes (1 can)

Dried thyme (½ teaspoon)

Dried rosemary (¼ teaspoon)

10. Water (2 cups)

Bay leaves (2 leaves)

Dried sage (½ teaspoon)

INSTRUCTIONS

1. Get a large pot and place it over medium heat. Drizzle in olive oil and stir fry garlic for about 1 minute.
2. Pour in carrots, celery and onion. Stir fry for 5 minutes or until vegetables are soft.
3. Stir in barley, sage, water, stock, bay leaves, tomatoes, rosemary and thyme. As soon as it boils, lower the heat and let the soup simmer for 45 minutes. If the barley isn't tender, leave it on to simmer a bit more.
4. Turn off the heat and remove all the leaves before serving.

Shrimp Cocktail Salad

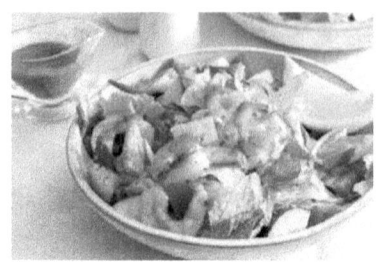

- Prep time: 10 minutes
- Cooking time: 5 minutes
- Serving: 4
- Calories: 163kcal
- Fats: 6g|Carbs: 4g|Protein: 17g

INGREDIENTS

1. Dried thyme (1 teaspoon)
2. Chopped romaine lettuce (1 large head)
3. Bay leaf (1 leaf)
4. Halved lemon with the seeds removed (1 medium)
5. Chopped cucumber, seeded (½ medium)
6. Black peppercorns (1 tablespoon)
7. Seafood sauce (⅓ cup)
8. Olive oil-based mayonnaise (¼ cup)
9. Unpeeled shrimp (1 pound)

Low-fat plain Greek yogurt (3 tablespoons)

INSTRUCTIONS

1. Pour water into a large pot until it is full. Squeeze some lemon juice into the pot and follow with thyme, bay leaf and peppercorns. The pot should be placed over high heat and left to boil.
2. Meanwhile, as the water boils, make your own ice bath. Pour water into a large bowl and toss in enough ice cubes. Set it aside
3. Throw the shrimp into the pot of boiling water and let them cook until they turn pink. This usually takes 2 or 3 minutes.
4. Get rid of the excess water by turning the shrimp into a colander. Now place the colander inside the ice bath and let it cool
5. As soon as it is cool enough to be touched, skin the shrimp and discard the tails.
6. Pour the yogurt, mayo and seafood sauce into a large bowl and whisk to mix thoroughly.
7. Pour the cooked skinless shrimp into the dressing and toss to coat.
8. Place lettuce on a plate, followed by cucumber and then the dressed shrimp.
9. Serve at once!

Tomato, Basil, And Cucumber Salad

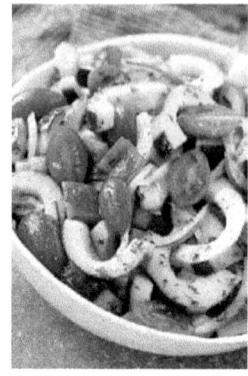

- Prep time: 15 minutes + 30 minutes
- Cooking time: 0
- Serving: 4
- Calories: 72kcal
- Fats: 4g | Carbs: 8g | Protein: 1g

INGREDIENTS

1. Red wine vinegar (3 tablespoons)
2. Sliced cucumber with the seeds removed (1 large)
3. Dijon mustard (½ teaspoon)
4. Thinly sliced red onion (1 medium)
5. Black pepper powder (½ teaspoon)
6. Quartered tomatoes (4 medium)
7. Finely chopped basil (½ cup)
8. Extra virgin olive oil (1 tablespoon)

INGREDIENTS

1. Throw tomatoes, basil, cucumber and red onion into a medium sized bowl and toss to mix.
2. Mix mustard, vinegar, pepper and olive oil in a much smaller bowl. Mix thoroughly and there! You made your dressing.
3. Now drizzle the dressing all over the veggies and toss to coat. Make sure you get some dressing on all the veggies
4. Put a lid on the bowl and place it in the refrigerator to cool for about 30 minutes.
5. Serve!

Notes: To make this simple salad a whole meal, grill a few pieces of chicken breast and dice them into bite sizes. Pour the chicken into the bowl of salad and toss to coat. This makes for a healthy and filling dinner or lunch.

Chapter 13: Tips For Eating Out

Imagine how nice it would be if we had the ability to wish fresh home-cooked meals into existence every night, especially on those very exhausting weekdays. This is definitely a goal for you to achieve. I understand that there will be days when you will dine at restaurants or at a friend's place, but you should do your best to keep this to a minimum.

It is advisable to relax for about 12 weeks after the procedure before you start eating outside your home, so you don't stray from your special diet. Also, you will need time to get used to your new lifestyle and your new stomach. You will need a few weeks to understand your tolerance and which foods to completely avoid. I have a list of tips to assist you in sticking to your new diet even when you're away from home:

Request for exactly what you would like. People always tend to forget that they're customers and have the right to make specific demands about what they would like as long as it is within the capacity of the seller. I mean, if you're at a restaurant you are paying for the meal and service. It is within your rights to ask as many questions as you like about the food and how it is made so you don't go eating what you shouldn't. Tell them you're currently on a special diet if you're comfortable with sharing that piece of information. A few hospitals give out special cards for this purpose just in case the patient isn't comfortable. Talk to your doctor about it.

Stick with steamed, grilled, broiled, poached and boiled foods. I'm sure you know by now that fried foods are definitely off limits. Don't even think about it. When you're eating out, ensure that you ask them if there is oil or extra butter in your food. You need to try as much as you can to eat home-cooked meals because most sauces prepared at restaurants usually have a high fat content or high sugar content. Avoid these for the sake of your weight and general health. Marinara and broth-based sauces are your best bets.

Do proper investigation. When making plans to eat at a restaurant or at someone else's home, I want you to understand how important it is to request the menu beforehand. A lot of restaurants these days have websites where they display their menus, so check them out first so you will know if you should eat at home or if it is safe to eat at the restaurant.

Feel free to carry your own food if it's allowed. It is very likely that you will have just a few bites and be instantly full, so just order something very small and simple like a shrimp cocktail or baked salmon.

Always be prepared even with family. If you have an occasion at a friend's place or a small party with family, go over your collection of safe recipes in this book and prepare something that is safe for you and is a crowd pleaser as well. This way, everybody wins, including your sleeve! You get to munch on something if your host doesn't have anything you can eat.

Good manners don't mean overeating. Request a doggie bag immediately you get served at the restaurant so that you don't get swamped with questions about why you aren't able to finish your food. You wouldn't want them to think the food is horrible or anything like that. Besides, I'd rather not have a plate half full of food staring me in the eyeball, would you? Exactly!

If you're with family or at a friend's place, request a to-go plate if they absolutely insist you have dessert or some other meal after you're sated. When you get home, you can decide to toss it, eat it later or hand it to someone else. Politeness doesn't require stuffing your face with foods you know you can't handle.

Conclusion

Vertical Sleeve Gastrectomy is more than just a bariatric procedure. It is a whole lot more. It is a journey that involves commitment, discipline, and a strength that I know you already possess. This comes with zero regrets, at least none I have heard of. This is a chance to feel alive again, to leave the shadows of your past behind. This book isn't and shouldn't be used as a substitute for professional advice, but it is all I can give and I assure you, it will be helpful even in the tiniest of ways.

When you do get started on this journey, make sure that you continue to educate yourself. Science keeps coming up with brand new things, and who knows which discovery may prove important to you on your VSG journey! You've got this, and you deserve the very best of health, happiness, and a wonderful, lithe, lean body. So go for it!

Remember, there will be some days when this is really tough, especially in the beginning. Be okay with that. Tell yourself it's only a bad day. That doesn't necessarily mean it has to be a bad life. One bad day is no excuse or reason to give up on your goals, or give in to your bad, old habits which never served you or your body. Besides, when you begin to see results, you will know deep down it was all worth it in the end. I'm rooting for you! Love and light.

Part 2

Introduction

As you probably know, there are four primary bariatric surgery procedures performed in the United States: a Roux-en-Y gastric bypass, a vertical gastrectomy sleeve (VSG), an adjustable gastric band, and a biliopancreatic bypass with a duodenal switch (BPD / DS). In 2013, the VSG has overtaken the Roux-en-Y gastric bypass as the most popular bariatric surgery in the United States.

The VSG as a unique weight-loss operation was originally the first part of a two-part bariatric surgery. Many surgeons conducted BPD / DS or gastric bypass as two consecutive procedures to reduce the risks associated with a prolonged procedure. Next, patients would have their stomach drained in an earlier, quicker, less risky operation— basically a sleeve gastrectomy.

Patients referred to the second part of the operation at a later date. Weight loss was so positive after the first phase of the treatment that some patients never returned to complete the second part of the operation. Therefore, the VSG was found to be a good weight-loss process with fewer risks than the other treatments with similar results.

Patients and providers love the gastrectomy of the sleeve. The procedure gained overwhelming popularity as a single weight-loss operation. The surgeon will remove three-fourths of the original stomach during this surgery. The banana-shaped stomach left behind is small, so it restricts the amount of food that a person can eat at any time.

During this process, no sensors are inserted. No modifications are made to any other portion of the intestinal tract of the human, which minimizes the possibility of long-term nutrient deficiencies. Throughout fact, the jacket produces great results when it comes to reducing comorbid ities, such as asthma and cardiovascular disease.

Chapter 1: Why Get Sleeved?

Choosing sleeve gastrectomy over other forms of bariatric surgery has many benefits. Here are some of the reasons why people are choosing to get sleeved.

1. Built-in segment power.

With only 15 to 25 percent of your stomach remaining following surgery, you are constrained in the amount of food you will consume at any given moment. You can still enjoy a variety of products with a change of food flavor post-op quality, but your stomach can give strong cues to let you know when you're finished and get you to stop eating.

2. Fewer pangs of hunger.

With the removal of the majority of the stomach, the hunger hormone ghrelin has decreased. Feeling less hunger supports reduced food intake.

3. Weight loss of more than half of your total body weight.

Excessive body weight is defined as any pound above your calculated ideal body weight for your height. Research reported by the American Society for Metabolic and Bariatric Surgery Integrated Health Nutritional Guidelines for Surgical Weight Loss Patients shows that people are able to maintain a weight loss of more than 55% of their excess body weight five years or more after surgery. For an individual who is 150 pounds in excess of their ideal weight, this means keeping at least 80 pounds off for the long term.

4. Eat candy with no wasting condition.

Many people have a hard time talking about giving up birthday cake or special-occasion ice cream for the rest of their lives following weight-loss surgery. Dumping syndrome is a disorder that may arise in individuals who have had gastric bypass or BPD / DS surgery after eating foods high in sugar and, in some instances, having too many carbs at one time.

Symptoms occur immediately after the meal in question and include a mixture of feeling nervous, light-headed, sweating or dizzy; elevated pulse rate; reduced blood sugar levels (reactive hypoglycemia); abdominal cramping; and diarrhea. Although large quantities of sweets may still cause dumping-like symptoms after VSG, it is very rare and not as severe as after weight-loss surgery, which involves the modification of the small intestine.

LESS TIME IN THE OPERATING ROOM

Any operation performed under general anesthesia involves risks and the potential for complications. These risks may multiply with the amount of time the operation takes to complete. Although the VSG is a longer treatment than the elastic brace, it is a quicker and easier method than the gastric bypass and the BPD / DS.

IF YOU CONSIDERING GASTRIC BYPASS

The main difference between the gastric bypass and the VSG is the second step of the gastric bypass process requiring the rerouting of the narrow intestinal tract. During the gastric bypass operation, a narrow cavity is developed from the wider stomach and part of the small intestinal tract is separated and attached to the new stomach.

To this end, the end side of the stomach and the upper part of the small intestinal tract are "deviated" during the digestion of food.

Similar to sleeve gastrectomy, gastric bypass produces slightly higher weight loss in the short term and slightly higher levels of type 2 diabetes resolution.

Dump syndrome may occur after gastric bypass when patients eat sweets. Dumping syndrome is often a good barrier to eating sweets for people struggling to minimize the calorie intake of sugary foods.

Another difference between gastric bypass and sleeve gastrectomy is that the gastric bypass immediately resolves any symptoms of gastroesophageal reflux disease or GERD after surgery. Following VSG, reflux can potentially get worse directly following surgery, but often improves with time. It is very important to discuss in depth the essence of your own behaviors and health history with your physician and medical team to decide which operation is better for you in the long term.

The recommendations for gastric bypass and VSG are very close when it comes to post-op care. You can still plan all the recipes for this book without having to worry over texture or section if you decide for a bypass.

Beginning with Nutrition A full team of medical professionals, comprising, at a minimum, a physician, a registered dietitian and a counselor, will help you better appreciate the operation as well as how to plan for it emotionally, psychologically and nutritionally.

But in the days, weeks, and years following surgery, success will depend on your ability to start with food in a real and lasting way. Part of this reset includes self-education in diet, and the other part requires self-management, which can be the hardest part of it.

CHALLENGES PEOPLE FACE AFTER SURGERY.

Embracing Food without Anxiety Through bariatric surgery, you decide to learn how to eat all over again. Beginning with only drinks, you can gradually move on to a balanced diet of almost all the food you might consume before surgery. You might be afraid to know just what's safe to eat, and you don't really want to eat again because of this anxiety.

In addition, you may be afraid of falling into old eating habits and losing the benefits of surgery. For accept food without doubt, concentrate on what you can consume instead of what you can't eat.

Stick to the basic principles of bariatric diet and choose to eat the food you know you can eat. It's going to take months for you to have complete confidence in your dos and don't have a bariatric diet, so give yourself time and don't try right away. If you stick to the rules for the first few weeks, you're not going to get sick. Time. Period. After that, listen to your body's messages.

Be patient and make every effort to stop eating at the first hint of fullness. Tap into your body's natural cues and stop taking another bite until you feel full. You don't have to live in fear; your body is going to tell you when to stop.

Come on to yourself. It's really different this time. You might be afraid to go back to the "old you" just like you used to die in the past. But now you've got the help of this beneficial surgery, which gives you a great start to your head. Now you're not just starting a diet, you're starting a whole lifestyle change: a permanent lifestyle change without turning back.

Recognize that support is of paramount importance. At least focus on your medical professionals, and hopefully at least a few associates, families, or colleagues. Turn to the people you trust to be encouraged when you feel scared. If you feel like you don't have anyone to support you, check again.

There's someone— a bariatric support group, a health coach, a psychologist, a pastor, a colleague. Talk with the one who can really motivate you through the bumps on the bridge. You become mentally and physically impaired from living in fear. Be assured that you can be effective in the post-op process and be aware of the choices you make every day.

CONTROLLING URGES

We've all got urges. Whether it's an impulse purchase at the mall, a second dessert help, or a wasteful day watching Netflix and a lack of workout— there are plenty of opportunities to give in and fall off your healthy lifestyle. The control of urges involves two parts.

1. Improve your mindfulness. Being mindful of your emotions, desires, and behavior in the present moment will help to curb your urges.

2. Don't give in to your cravings. For some individuals, giving in to temptation involves flipping a key, putting it back into an "on" role that might have been blocked. How many times does eating a chip turn into half a bag, drinking a glass of wine into half a bottle, or eating an Oreo turn into a whole sleeve? For many bariatric patients, giving in to desires, compulsions, or impulses can contribute to binge-type behavior.

Practice awareness and remind yourself if this is what the body actually needs at the moment. Sometimes the reaction is "yeah," that's just what you need. Yet stop and ask again before giving in to a slight impulse, as it often adds to a domino effect in self-harming habits.

DEMONSTRATING SELF-COMPASSION

What we act about ourselves and what we handle ourselves for good and bad attitudes directly affects our satisfaction. It can also affect our ability to keep up with long-term behavioral changes following surgery. The doctor describes self-compassion as three parts— self-kindness, empathy, and common humanity.

During treatment, both patients make mistakes. It's whether we react with self-compassion or self-criticism that defines how strong we are after a time of slipping back into old habits. We are all individual, and we have our own imperfections. Take advantage of your good qualities and accept your challenges, too.

Seek to use your talents to solve challenges in other fields. Self-denigration is only going to move you farther further from your ambitions. When you've got a couple of bad days, realize that your subconscious might have needed a break.

Try to move forward without focusing too much on past mistakes, and look forward to your continued success.

APPRECIATING NATURAL SWEETNESS

We live in a culture where our threshold for sweetness is growing higher and higher. Desserts are growing increasingly natural and soft beverages are becoming sweeter. Changing the habit of eating candy can be especially difficult for anyone trying to lose weight because sugar is addictive.

Eating sugary snacks turns your brain's pleasure centers light, causing you want to go out for more. If this is something you've been struggling with, bariatric surgery gives you the chance to press the reset button. You're going to get a redo on your food preferences and an opportunity to get some major help in pushing old habits to the edge.

Focus on eating naturally sweet food to balance your need to satisfy all taste buds. Include grains such as barley or quinoa, which have a sweet and nutty flavor and are still packed with plenty of nutrients. Instead of sugary desserts, top off your meal with something naturally sweet like fresh berries or fresh citrus fruits

Even using 100% cocoa powder in protein shakes or other baked goods, you can reduce your chocolate cravings without extra sugar and fat from typical milk chocolate candies. Appreciating the natural sweetness of food will help to put down the sugar addiction!

MANAGING WEIGHT — Management EXPECTATIONS

Weight loss is not a perfect science. Even in a controlled weight-loss study, there is still some variation in the weight loss of individuals. It's hard to send you a 110 percent commitment, and the outcomes aren't what you expect. To order to manage the post-op weight loss goals, don't put undue strain on yourself to lose weight more rapidly than is practical. Okay, learn yourself. Others may lose weight faster or slower than you do.

The causes that lead in weight loss are multifaceted and some are out of your influence. Did you know that weight loss might even affect the amount of sleep you get? In addition to food intake, exercise, muscle mass, stress, starting body weight, height, gender, age, and even more factors all play a part in the amount of weight you lose. Be vigilant, and polite, and don't equate yourself with others.

Your weight-loss path is unique; it's all right and you're going to be disappointed at times. Just know that you will achieve long-term success with continued hard work.

ENJOYING FOOD AGAIN

During the first few days of post-op, when you consume mostly liquids, it's hard to imagine that you'll ever find pleasure in eating food again. Initially, it can be a chore, something done out of necessity.

Questions can begin to flutter: can I look forward to eating again? Will I ever be able to eat the food I used to love?

Keep in mind that right after surgery, your body undergoes rapid physical and hormonal changes— all of which suppress your urge to eat and the amount you can eat.

Most of your initial rapid weight loss is the result of a combination of these changes. Be patient with me. When time progresses, you will be comfortable and able to eat a slightly larger amount of food and accept a wider variety of foods.

I know this may sound untrue, but some people who really enjoyed pizza and ice cream before surgery may no longer want to consume certain kinds of food. When you move on to a diet full of nutritious foods and leaving aside high-calorie foods, you will notice that your body is more ready for healthier foods. And this is the best time to try some of your favorite old recipes— with a safer twist.

Food is food for your body; it's a must to feed every single day. Yet mealtime is so much more than what we place in our mouths. With a little preparation, flexibility, and willingness to experiment, it's really possible to enjoy nutritious food after surgery.

FREQUENTLY ASKED QUESTIONS

After surgery, stay connected to your bariatric medical team and support group so that you can easily get answers to your questions and concerns from a reliable source— and receive support and encouragement. Here are a few questions that I have frequently been asked.

Taking a walk down the nutrition and vitamin row in your grocery store may be daunting. There are hundreds of products on the market, each of which promises to be different than the next. You want to set a strong diet plan because you're not going to drink protein shakes for the rest of your life. Protein shakes and powders should be a bridge for the first few days and weeks to allow you to eat whole foods. In comparison, protein powders can be used to help you easily take in a rich source of high-quality protein with very few calories. Here are my guidelines for bariatric-friendly protein powder.

Choose the protein whey isolate. It's easier for your body to absorb, and it's dense in essential amino acids. Other high quality sources include soya protein (vegan) isolates or egg white powders.

Use some unflavored protein powder. We are low in calories and the cleanest since they are safe from artificial ingredients.

Use sugar-free with flavored protein powders

Okay, look for completely sugar-free varieties that are sweetened with stevia, sucralose (Splenda) or other sugar substitutes. There are hundreds of taste choices from coffee to pecan oil, so you'll be pleased with very few calories. Sugar substitutes are FDA-approved, calorie-free, and healthy to use after surgery.

Be vigilant of sugar alcohols (erythritol, mannitol, xylitol, and sorbitol) because they add calories and may induce unwanted gastrointestinal side effects.

Find the sample sizes you need to try before your surgery. Search for free or discounted products on the manufacturer's website. This way, you'll realize what you like and what you don't have in order for the first few days of post-op.

Get something quick and easy, such as low-fat cottage cheese or Greek yogurt, hard-boiled eggs, nitrate-free turkey or chicken lunch meat or low-fat cheese. Milk or protein shake may also fulfill the protein target. The key is to focus on hitting your protein target at least 80% of the time. Begin the next day with a high-protein breakfast to make up for what you might have lost the day before.

It seems impossible that eating straight protein foods for weeks and months to come could be considered a healthy lifestyle, but it's only temporary. The multivitamin should mask what you're going to lose of nutrients during this process. Work on making it a priority to consume fruit and vegetables as the first items you choose once you're able to spread past proteins.

Various types of fruit and vegetables throughout the week since it's hard to eat a few portions in a single day. There are hundreds of recipes in this book that give tips on how to slip fruit and vegetables right into your main protein dishes. Work your way up to five servings of fruit and vegetables a day in the long run.

There are two specific reasons why people do not eat doughy bread products and pasta following surgery. The first is that the current stomach is not well handled. The sleeve has a hard time digesting these foods in the first few months. If you eat them, you may feel overly full quickly and then hungry shortly after, or you may feel bloated, and/or you may feel that something is stuck in your small stomach.

Such symptoms usually arise after the first few months, but some people experience pain from consuming such types of foods over the longer term. The second reason people restrict carbohydrate intake is to rely more on consuming protein foods for fullness and fruits and vegetables that are low in calories. It's not bad to eat bread and pasta following surgery if you can handle it — it should be mild, concentrating first on nutrition, then fruits, then carbs.

It's ideal to enlist the support of loved ones, partners, family, and friends before surgery, but you can't always wait to change your lifestyle until everyone you know is equally ready. Here are a few tips to stay on track when the rest of the household might be more resistant.

Hold the most enticing remedies out of the pantry. Allow only the convenient rewards that you can avoid. Oreos may be your greatest weakness, but the rest of the household couldn't care less if the cookies were Chips Ahoy or Nutter Butters. Don't buy Oreos, but let family favorites do not tempt you.

Figure out the source. Whether it's heading out for a stroll, going to bed early, getting lost in a good book, or texting a friend — find an outlet for pain, fear, or depression that's not eating. Make sure you have an alternate option for yourself when your name is called by the potato chips.

Have simple meals on hand for yourself and the rest of your family. Make every effort to stop becoming a short-term post-op chef. Have some food on hand so there's always something safe, simple, and easy going around. When appropriate, consider foods that can be quickly changed to suit your needs and the taste preferences of others.

Tell about what you need. Not everyone in the family will appreciate the wishes while you adopt a bariatric diet. Practice good communication and make sure you know what you need for support. You can't assume that other people know what your objectives are and what you need to do.

Weight-loss surgery is a procedure on your chest, but it does not alter the pre-operative eating habits in your head. With that in mind, I strongly suggest that patients establish as many healthy and positive eating patterns ahead of time with a post-op diet in mind. Keeping the patterns in order before treatment will make things a lot easier when you're healing.

It's overwhelming to ask yourself how to count protein grams, give up fast food, stop drinking liquids with food, and start taking multivitamin supplements all at once. Whether or not the surgical center needs you to adopt a pre-operative regimen of some kind is independent of your preference to develop as many post-op routines as practicable in advance of time.

Most bariatric surgery plans and/or insurance companies include some kind of pre-operative weight loss, high-protein diet, or liquid diet within days, weeks, and sometimes months before surgery. Losing weight in the last week or two before surgery, particularly through a low-carbohydrate or liquid diet, can help to reduce the size of the liver and lower abdominal fat, making surgery simpler for the surgeon and healthier for you.

Just Keep Trying When you wake up from bariatric surgery, your entire lifestyle will only change if you choose to make it different. Surgery doesn't prohibit you from eating fast food. Surgery doesn't allow you get out of the sofa. Surgery doesn't stop you from having a bag of potato chips every dinner.

Modifying a century of behaviors to meet your weight loss goals can be difficult. Although you're going to face hurdles and challenges, just keep trying. Babies don't learn how to run before they can walk about. So just do these small things. You may only be able to walk for 10 minutes without getting exhausted, but 10 minutes is a start.

You may not be able to give up candy entirely, but you can mix in smaller portions. You may not be able to give up fast food, but you can get a burger without a side of the fries. Small steps are making a difference. Set realistic, attainable goals for yourself. You're going to have weeks when the pounds fall off in double digits, and weeks when you don't seem to be making the scale budge. Don't give it up. Don't lose your hope. Just keep on trying. Keep a food log for a couple of days. Try a new kind of fitness class. Go to bed 30 minutes earlier to get some extra sleep. Schedule a follow-up to your bariatric medical team. Just keep on trying.

ALCOHOL AFTER VSG

When you had a few alcoholic beverages before bariatric surgery, and you're curious if this is something you should proceed with after treatment, you should have a good understanding of how the operation will impact the absorption of alcohol. There is an enzyme in the stomach that helps partially digest alcohol. Since most of the stomach is eliminated during VSG, the capacity to break down alcohol will be significantly altered.

As a consequence, even a tiny amount of alcohol consumption is highly intoxicating. The smaller body size and limited food intake will also lead to alcohol intoxication and dehydration. Moreover, alcohol is extremely dense in calories. Bariatric surgery does not restrict liquid calories, and alcohol calories can add up very quickly.

Weddings, family gatherings, parties— alcohol can be a major part of socializing, but for many post-op patients, alcohol intake can be a replacement for food as an outlet from pain. According to the Obesity Action Coalition, the likelihood of relapse following bariatric surgery is increased due to something called a transition of addiction. People trade drug consumption as an escape for pain, sadness, or anxiety. And think twice before drinking champagne following surgery — think about making yourself a designated driver and go for non-alcoholic drinks instead.

When drinking is a problem for you or your loved one, realize that your bariatric medical team is there to serve you; assistance is waiting for you. Alcoholism is not supposed to be kept hidden, and you are not alone. You can also find information about Alcoholics Anonymous in the Resources section of this report.

Alcoholics Anonymous can help you determine if you have a problem with the transfer of addiction and help you fight it.

Chapter 2: Breakfast

Southwestern Scrambled Egg Burritos

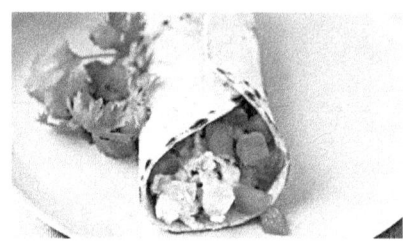

PREP TIME: 10 MINUTES

COOK TIME: 10 MINUTES

TOTAL TIME: 20 MINUTES

SERVINGS: 8

These breakfast burritos have the ingredients you crave but without all the added sodium and fat. Make them freeze and then toss one in the microwave for a hot breakfast in minutes.

INGREDIENTS

- 12 eggs
- ¼ cup low-fat milk
- 1 teaspoon extra-virgin olive oil
- ½ onion, chopped
- 1 red bell pepper, diced
- 1 green bell pepper, diced

- 1 (15-ounce) can black beans, drained and rinsed
- 8 (7- to 8-inch) whole-wheat tortillas, such as La Tortilla Factory low-carb tortillas
- 1 cup salsa, for serving

PREPARATIONS

Using a big bowl stir the eggs and milk. Set aside.

In a large skillet over medium-high heat, heat the olive oil and add the onion and bell peppers. Sauté for 2 to 3 minutes, or until tender. Add the beans and stir to combine.

Add the egg mixture. Minimize heat and mix while constantly with a rubber spatula for 5 minutes, until the eggs are fluffy and cooked through.

Divide the scrambled egg mixture among the tortillas. Fold over the bottom end of the tortilla, fold in the sides, and roll tightly to close.

Serve immediately with the salsa, or place each burrito in a zip-top bag and refrigerate for up to 1 week. To eat, reheat each burrito in the microwave for 60 to 90 seconds. These will also keep well in the freezer for up to 1 month.

Serving tip: To get more vegetables into your breakfast, buy a bag of frozen California-blend mixed vegetables. Heat some in a skillet with extra-virgin olive oil, add eggs, and—voilà!—a quick veggie-packed egg burrito.

NUTRITIONAL VALUE

Per Serving (1 burrito): Calories: 250; Total fat: 10g; Protein: 19g; Carbs: 28g; Fiber: 13g; Sugar: 1g; Sodium: 546mg

Smoothie Bowl With Greek Yogurt And Fresh Berries

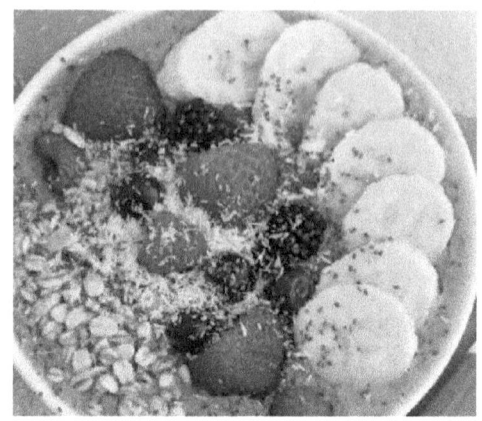

PREP TIME: 5 MINUTES

COOK TIME: 5 MINUTES

TOTAL TIME: 10 MINUTES

SERVINGS: 1

The appearance of our food and where we eat our meals can strongly affect our feelings of satiety after eating. In fact, after surgery, whether you're eating in a high-stress environment or having a relaxing candlelit dinner can influence whether a food makes you sick. Instead of slamming a protein shake for your next breakfast on the way out the door, try sitting down to enjoy this refreshing smoothie bowl. It is just as appealing to the eye as the stomach. Slow down and savor every bite of this smoothie you can eat with a spoon!

INGREDIENTS

- ¾ cup unsweetened vanilla almond milk or low-fat milk
- ¼ cup low-fat plain Greek yogurt
- ⅓ cup (1 handful) fresh spinach
- ½ scoop (⅛ cup) plain or vanilla protein powder
- ¼ cup frozen mixed berries
- ¼ cup fresh raspberries
- ¼ cup fresh blueberries
- 1 tablespoon sliced, slivered almonds
- 1 teaspoon chia seeds

PREPARATION

In a blender, combine the milk, yogurt, spinach, protein powder, and frozen berries. For 4 minutes blend, until the powder is well dissolved and no longer visible.

Pour the smoothie into small bowl.

Decorate the smoothie with the fresh raspberries, blueberries, almonds, and chia seeds.

Serve with a spoon and enjoy!

Serving tip: You can make this smoothie bowl with a variety of other fruits and toppings to change it up. Try a mango-pineapple version. Top with unsweetened, flaked coconut and use coconut milk in the smoothie base for a more tropical vibe.

NUTRITIONAL VALUE

Per Serving (1 bowl): Calories: 255; Total fat: 10 g; Protein: 20g; Carbs: 21g; Fiber: 8g; Sugar: 10g; Sodium: 262mg

Cherry-Vanilla Baked Oatmeal

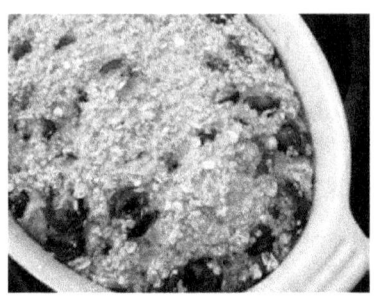

PREP TIME: 10 MINUTES

COOK TIME: 45 MINUTES

TOTAL TIME: 55 MINUTES

SERVINGS: 6

Look no farther than this baked oatmeal recipe to replace your run-of-the-mill coffee shop pastry—the ones that are high in sugar, high in fat, and high in calories. The sweet flavor and hearty ingredients of this baked oatmeal will leave you feeling warm and satisfied on any cold winter morning. Bake for Sunday breakfast and eat leftovers throughout the week.

INGREDIENTS

- Nonstick cooking spray
- 1 cup old-fashioned oats
- ½ teaspoon ground cinnamon
- ¾ teaspoon baking powder
- 1 tablespoon ground flaxseed
- 3 eggs
- 1 cup low-fat milk
- ½ cup low-fat plain Greek yogurt

- 1 teaspoon vanilla extract
- 1 teaspoon liquid stevia (optional; to improve sweetness)
- 1 cup fresh pitted cherries
- 1 apple, peeled, cored and chopped

PREPARATION

Preheat the oven to 375°F. Lightly coat an 8-by-8-inch baking dish with the cooking spray.

Mix together the oats, cinnamon, baking powder, and flaxseed in a medium bowl. In a separate large bowl, gently whisk the eggs, milk, yogurt, vanilla, and stevia (if using).

Combine the dry ingredients and mix to combine. Gently fold in the cherries and apples.

Bake for 45 minutes or until the edges start to pull away from the side of the pan and the oatmeal gently bounces back when touched.

Divide leftover oatmeal into airtight glass containers. Refrigerate for up to 1 week for quick and easy breakfast, or freeze.

Serving tip: Experiment with the fixings in your baked oatmeal. I like to make my recipes seasonal. Replace the yogurt with pumpkin puree to add a hint of fall. Try using unsweetened dried cranberries instead of cherries for a holiday twist. Swap out apples and cherries for 2 cups fresh berries in spring for a very berry oatmeal! For the creamiest consistency, I recommend topping with a ¼ cup low-fat milk at serving time.

NUTRITIONAL VALUE

Per Serving (½ cup): Calories: 149; Total fat: 4g; Protein: 8g; Carbs: 21g; Fiber: 4g; Sugar: 9g; Sodium: 71 mg

High-Protein Pancakes

PREP TIME: 5 MINUTES

COOK TIME: 5 MINUTES

TOTAL TIME: 10 MINUTES

SERVINGS: 4

Try these high-protein pancakes this weekend. Made with simple ingredients already in your pantry and refrigerator, these hotcakes are sure to be a crowd pleaser.

INGREDIENTS

- 3 eggs
- 1 cup low-fat cottage cheese
- ⅓ cup whole-wheat pastry flour
- 1½ tablespoons coconut oil, melted
- Nonstick cooking spray

PREPARATIONS

In large bowl, lightly whisk the eggs.

Whisk in the cottage cheese, flour, and coconut oil just until combined.

Heat a large skillet or griddle over medium heat, and lightly coat with the cooking spray.

Using a measuring cup, pour ⅓ cup of batter into the skillet for each pancake, Boil   for 3 minutes and till bubbles appear across the surface of each pancake

Flip over the pancakes and cook for 1 to 2 minutes on the other side, or until golden brown.

Serve immediately.

Serving tip: Top these pancakes with fresh berries and plain yogurt, unsweetened applesauce, or sugar-free syrup. You can even try them with natural peanut butter and bananas on a general diet.

NUTRITIONAL VALUE

Per Serving (1 pancake): Calories: 182; Total fat: 10g; Protein: 12g; Carbs: 10g; Fiber: 3g; Sugar: 1g; Sodium: 68mg

Pumpkin Muffins With Walnuts And Zucchini

PREP TIME: 10 MINUTES

COOK TIME: 25 MINUTES

TOTAL TIME: 35 MINUTES

SERVINGS: 4

Most muffins you pick up at your local bakery are packed with loads of sugar, white flour, and plenty of fat. Luckily, it's easy to make your own soft and delicious muffins at home with a few healthy twists. These muffins stay light and moist because they are made with shredded zucchini and pureed pumpkin.

INGREDIENTS

- Nonstick cooking spray or baking liners
- 2 cups old-fashioned oats
- 1¾ cups whole-wheat pastry flour
- ¼ cup ground flaxseed
- 2 tablespoons baking powder
- 1 teaspoon baking soda
- 1 teaspoon ground cinnamon
- ¼ teaspoon ground nutmeg
- ¼ teaspoon ground ginger
- ¼ teaspoon ground allspice
- 2 cups shredded zucchini
- 1 cup canned pumpkin or fresh pumpkin puree
- 1 cup low-fat milk
- 4 eggs, lightly beaten
- ¼ cup unsweetened applesauce
- 1 teaspoon liquid stevia
- ½ cup chopped walnuts

PREPARATIONS

Preheat the oven to 375°F. Prepare two muffin tins by coating the cups with the cooking spray, or use baking liners.

In large bowl, mix together the oats, flour, flaxseed, baking powder, baking soda, cinnamon, nutmeg, ginger, and allspice.

In a separate medium bowl mix together the zucchini, pumpkin, milk, eggs, applesauce, and stevia

Add the wet ingredients to the dry and stir to combine. Gently stir in the walnuts.

Fill the cups of the muffin tins about half full with the batter.

Bake until the muffins are done, when a toothpick inserted in the center comes out clean, about 25 minutes.

Let the muffins cool for 5 minutes before removing them from the tins. Place on a baking rack to finish cooling.

Wrap leftover muffins in plastic wrap and freeze. Reheat frozen muffins in the microwave for about 20 seconds.

Ingredient tip: Put the shredded zucchini in a colander in the sink and press it with the back of a spoon to drain the moisture; pat dry with paper towels before adding to the bowl.

Did You Know? Flaxseed is rich in omega-3s. Omega-3 fats have anti-inflammatory effects in the body and may help promote a healthy brain and healthy heart. Ground flaxseed is also a great source of fiber. It can be mixed into smoothies, cereal, or yogurt. It can also be easily added to baked goods. Swap out ¼ cup of flour for ¼ cup of ground flaxseed in any baking recipe to get more of this nutrient-packed seed into your diet!

NUTRITIONAL VALUE

Per Serving (1 muffin): Calories: 128; Total fat: 5g; Protein: 5g; Carbs: 18g; Fiber: 3g; Sugar: 1g; Sodium: 86mg

Hard-Boiled Eggs And Avocado On Toast

PREP TIME: 10 MINUTES

COOK TIME: 10 MINUTES

TOTAL TIME: 20 MINUTES

SERVINGS: 4

A diet staple after a sleeve gastrectomy, eggs are packed with protein, vitamins, and minerals. Eggs are rich in choline, which is essential for brain and liver function. Choose organic free-range eggs when possible, as their yolks contain more heart-healthy omega-3 fats than conventional versions. Hard-boil a dozen eggs at a time and keep them on hand to eat throughout the week.

INGREDIENTS

- 4 eggs
- 4 slices sprouted whole-wheat bread, such as Angelic Bakehouse Sprouted Grain
- 1 medium avocado
- 1 teaspoon hot sauce
- Freshly ground black pepper
-

PREPARATIONS

Using a pot fill it up and rapid boil over high heat.

Carefully add the eggs to the boiling water using a spoon, and set a timer for 10 minutes.

Immediately transfer the eggs from the boiling water to a strainer, and run cold water over the eggs to stop the cooking process.

Once the eggs are cool enough to handle, peel them and slice lengthwise into fourths.

Toast the bread.

While the bread toasts, mash the avocado with a fork in a small bowl and mix in the hot sauce.

Spread the avocado mash evenly across each toast. Top each toast slice with 4 egg slices and season with the black pepper.

Ingredient tip: Avocado is rich in healthy fat, but also loaded with calories, so portion control is key. Store the pit with any unused portion of avocado, squeeze a teaspoon of lemon juice over the leftovers, and place in an airtight container or wrap in plastic wrap to prevent browning.

NUTRITIONAL VALUE

Per Serving (1 toast): Calories: 191; Total fat: 10g; Protein: 10g; Carbs: 15g; Fiber: 5g; Sugar: 1g; Sodium: 214mg

Chapter 3: Vegetarian Dinners

Mexican Stuffed Summer Squash

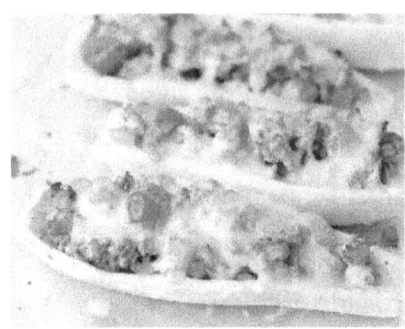

PREP TIME: 5 MINUTES

COOK TIME: 33 MINUTES

TOTAL TIME: 38 MINUTES

SERVINGS: 2

Here is a great low-carb dish that will satisfy your cravings and use some of summer's most plentiful vegetables. It's easy enough to double or triple to make for a family or for you to eat throughout the week.

INGREDIENTS

- Nonstick cooking spray
- 1 yellow summer squash
- ½ cup Refried Black Beans or canned fat-free refried pinto beans with 1 teaspoon taco seasoning mixed in (for flavor)
- ½ cup cooked quinoa

- ¼ cup shredded Colby Jack cheese
- 1 small tomato, diced
- 2 tablespoons sliced black olives
- 2 scallions, chopped, for garnish

PREPARATIONS

Preheat the oven to 400°F. Coat an 8-by-8-inch baking dish with the cooking spray.

Cut the ends off of the summer squash and discard. Cut lengthwise, then use a spoon to remove and discard the seeds. Place the squash halves cut-side down in the baking dish. Gently poke a couple of holes in the squash to vent. Add 1 tablespoon of water to the dish. Microwave for about 3 minutes or until slightly tender. Discard any leftover water.

When cool enough to handle, turn the squash so they are skin-side down and spaced evenly apart in the dish.

Layer ¼ cup of the beans in each squash, then ¼ cup of the quinoa, Top the whole thing with the Colby Jack cheese. Cover with aluminum foil and bake for 25 minutes. Remove the foil and bake for 5 minutes more, or until the cheese is bubbly and the squash is tender.

Garnish each squash with the tomatoes, olives, and scallions just before serving.

Serving tip: Get creative with extras. Brown ground turkey or a soy-based meat substitute in taco seasoning and add on top of the beans. Sauté bell peppers and onions to layer on or serve with avocado and cilantro

NUTRITIONAL VALUE

Per Serving (1 squash half): Calories: 190; Total fat: 8 g; Protein: 9g; Carbs: 21g; Fiber: 4g; Sugar: 3g; Sodium: 40mg

Roasted Vegetable Quinoa Salad With Chickpeas

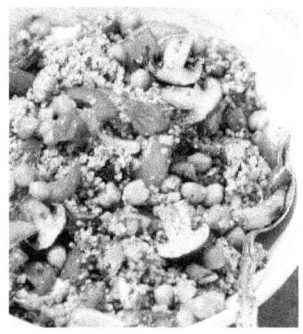

PREP TIME: 15 MINUTES

COOK TIME: 30 MINUTES

TOTAL TIME: 45 MINUTES

SERVINGS: 6

Many people find that their sleeve tolerates cooked vegetables better than raw vegetables in the initial months post-op. This quinoa salad is an excellent alternative to traditional lettuce salads. It contains a variety of vegetarian protein sources— quinoa and chickpeas—and it's loaded with vegetables that have been roasted to bring out their natural rich flavors.

INGREDIENTS

- 1 small eggplant, diced
- 1 small zucchini, diced
- 1 small yellow summer squash, diced
- ½ cup grape tomatoes, halved
- 1 (15-ounce) can chickpeas, drained and rinsed
- 3 tablespoons extra-virgin olive oil, divided

- ⅓ cup packaged quinoa
- 1 cup low-sodium vegetable or chicken broth
- 2 tablespoons freshly squeezed lemon juice
- 1 teaspoon minced fresh garlic or 1 garlic clove, minced
- 1 tablespoon dried basil
- 1 teaspoon dried oregano

PREPARATIONS

Preheat the oven to 425°F. Line a 9-by-13-inch baking sheet with parchment paper.

Spread the eggplant, zucchini, yellow squash, tomatoes, and chickpeas across the baking sheet and toss them with 1 tablespoon of olive oil.

Bake for 30 minutes, stirring once halfway through. The finished vegetables should be tender and the tomatoes should be juicy. The chickpeas will be firm and crispy.

While the vegetables and chickpeas are roasting, place the quinoa and broth in a small saucepan over medium-high heat. Cover and bring to a boil. Minimize heat and boil for about 15 minutes, or until all liquid has absorbed. Remove the pan from the heat and fluff the quinoa with a fork. (Otherwise, make the quinoa according to the package instructions.)

In a small dish, whisk together the lemon juice, garlic, and remaining 2 tablespoons of olive oil. Mix in the basil and oregano.

Using a big bowl mix the quinoa, roasted vegetables with chickpeas, and dressing. Gently stir to combine. Serve and enjoy!

Serving tip: To increase the protein in this dish, you can add lean grilled chicken breast or serve with a piece of baked fish. You can always top with a dollop of low-fat plain Greek yogurt.

NUTRITIONAL VALUE

Per Serving (½ cup): Calories: 200; Total fat: 9g; Protein: 7g; Carbs: 27g; Fiber: 8g; Sugar: 4g; Sodium: 160mg

www.ingramcontent.com/pod-product-compliance
Lightning Source LLC
Chambersburg PA
CBHW071442070526
44578CB00001B/199